KAPLAN® ...we'll t[barcode] e.

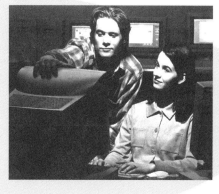
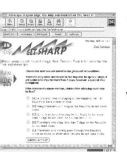

Let Kaplan Be Your Guide...
Books and Software to Help You
Reach Your Educational Goals.

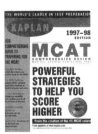

Score Higher!
Maximize your performance on test day with expert advice for the GRE, GMAT, LSAT and MCAT.

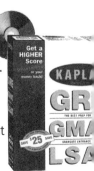

Pick the Study Method
That's Right For You.
Kaplan offers you its proven methods in the format you prefer—whether it be books or software.

Get Expert Admissions and Financial Aid Advice.
Information packed guides for college and graduate school admissions, featuring insider's advice on everything from writing effective essays to finding ways to help pay for your education.

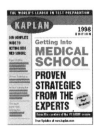
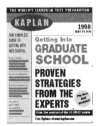
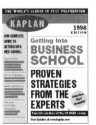
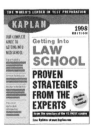

Available at bookstores and software outlets everywhere.
For more information, call 1-800-KAP-ITEM.

NO POSTAGE
NECESSARY
IF MAILED
IN THE
UNITED STATES

BUSINESS REPLY MAIL
FIRST CLASS MAIL   PERMIT NO. 2479   NEW YORK, NY

POSTAGE WILL BE PAID BY ADDRESSEE

KAPLAN
P.O. BOX 9112
MEDFORD, NY 11763-9940

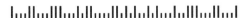

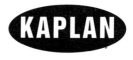

Kaplan Books Relating to Medical School Admissions

Getting into Medical School 1998
MCAT 1997–98
MCAT Comprehensive Review 1997–98

Other Books in This Series

The Insider's Book of Business School Lists
The Insider's Book of Law School Lists

THE INSIDER'S BOOK OF MEDICAL SCHOOL LISTS

by Mark Baker

Simon & Schuster

Kaplan Books
Published by Kaplan Educational Centers and Simon & Schuster
1230 Avenue of the Americas
New York, NY 10020

Manufactured in the United States of America
Published Simultaneously in Canada

August 1997

10 9 8 7 6 5 4 3 2 1

The data in this book is subject to frequent change. Every attempt was made to
ensure that all figures were current at the time this book went to press.

The author thanks Frank Fortunato, Robyn English Turner, and Ron Green for
their research, wit, and gracious cooperation; and Lee Rinaldo of Sonic Youth
and Joe Woodard for their expert input on music and culture.

Special thanks are extended to Linda Volpano, Sara Pearl, Rochelle Rothstein,
M.D., Richard Friedland, D.P.M., William Dracos, and Andrew Taylor.

Project Editor: Richard Christiano
Production Coordinator: Gerard Capistrano
Production Editor: Maude Spekes
Interior Design/Production: gumption design
Cover Design: Amy McHenry
Assistant Managing Editor: Brent Gallenberger
Managing Editor: Kiernan McGuire
Executive Editor: Del Franz

ISSN: 1093-1449
ISBN: 0-684-84178-9

CONTENTS

INTRODUCTION

So, you've made it through 12 years of basic education, at least four years of college, and now you're on the verge of mortgaging the ranch for four more years of textbooks, lectures, all-nighters, weekends in the library instead of on the beach, and the daily certainty of having a pop quiz in your life. By continuing your studies in medical school, you've committed yourself to one of the most demanding, stressful, pressurized lifestyles in America today, perhaps rivaled only by deep-sea diving underwater welders and air traffic controllers. Right now, it looks like a long, hard road rolling out in front of you toward infinity. You've probably narrowed your choices down to three or four schools that fit your credentials, your special talents, and your budget. If you're like most medical school candidates, you've filled out a mountain of forms. You've spent countless hours polishing and updating your personal essay, trying to walk that incredibly thin line between sucking up and stuck up. Then there's the begging for letters of recommendation and the awful fear that some professor, employer, or family physician is suddenly going to go psycho on you and have you blackballed globally. You've struggled to prepare for interviews with a bunch of total strangers, and then stammered through the ordeal wondering what in the world they mean with their secret code of winks, coughs, and foot shuffling.

What you want most—more than another Cross pen and pencil set—is just a little break from the pressure cooker: a change of perspective, a couple of laughs. That's where *The Insider's Book of Medical School Lists* comes in.

These lists put the next few years of grueling higher education into a broader, more worldly context. There's more to life than going to class. What about surfing, shopping, and rock-and-roll? What about the ratio of days of sunshine to days of rain, convenient spring break resorts, famous and infamous alumni? What about roller coasters, golf, and nightclubs? And there's more to education than just lectures, projects, and tests. What about great overseas programs, cheap-o application fees, and flexible classroom hours? Which schools have the most eligible women, and which have the most eligible men?

We would never suggest that you make a final decision about which institution of higher learning to set your heart upon simply by referring to our list of schools on the Lollapalooza Tour. It wouldn't be right to decide to attend a medical school just because it was located within 30 minutes of great skiing. No one in his right mind would pick a graduate school just because it was near some of the best microbreweries in the nation. Right?

On the other hand, these details of life and education are not to be sniffed at. You've worked really hard to get where you are today—teetering on the brink of four more years of even harder work—so maybe it wouldn't be such a bad idea to include the Fun Factor in your equation for the perfect medical school. Passion in life is a good thing. So what if your passion is for mall crawling and lounge lizards? If you're going to do your best in medical school, you need an outlet for your extracurricular passions, you've got to keep in touch with real life beyond the halls of academe. And you need a school that will help you claw your way to the top, instead of ripping you to shreds.

A few of the lists compiled in the following pages are strictly serious, some are seriously silly, and a few are strictly for laughs. You could probably use a good laugh about now. So plow right in and read cover to cover, or use the index to choose the subjects you want to investigate further or the schools you'd like to know more about. However you choose to absorb this essential information about your future, be sure to relax and enjoy yourself.

GETTING IN
AND STAYING IN

PART 1

"Imagine walking into a room occupied by 35 tiny and very sick premature newborn babies. For the nest 12 hours, their well being, their very survival is your responsibility. That was how my internship year began. It was definitely one of the most terrifying days of my life.

"I somehow survived that year in spite of the fact that I and the other interns in my group received negligible guidance from the senior people in the program. I was overworked, overtired, lonely and insecure, often depressed, and conflicted by my own responsibilities, whether admitting an infant with a dangerously high fever or coping with the psychological and physical stresses of dealing with AIDS patients.

"My internship was the hardest, most devastating year of my life. It's been eight and a half years since I finished that year and some of the pain, the anger, the exhaustion, and the anguish is still with me.

"When the intern learns about medicine and the human body, he or she truly becomes a physician. But in the process, through the wearing down of the intern's spirit, that person loses something he or she has carried, some innocence, some humanness, some fundamental respect. The question is, 'Is it all worth it?'"

—Robert Marion, M.D.
The Intern Blues
Ballantine, 1989

There are plenty of theories about how to choose the best medical school. There's the Academic Theory, which insists that the toughest school with the highest academic standards is the only logical choice. There's the Status Theory, which posits that your future will be assured only if you attend a medical school with a national reputation for its credentials. If you subscribe to the You Get What You Pay For Theory, then only the most expensive graduate school will do. Those are only a few of the more prominent theories.

The Insider's Book of Medical School Lists just doesn't buy any of them. They all have their place, and perhaps some merit. But they all concentrate on the schools and leave you, the prospective student, out of the equation. If you're going to do your best in medical school, and you want an institution that will nurture your success, fulfill your dreams, and guarantee your future, then the first thing to do is look at what *you* want—your likes and dislikes, your strengths and foibles.

Just for a change, let's concentrate on what will make you happy. What sort of working conditions will make you comfortable? How much are you willing to pay? What kind of a crowd will you be hanging with in this joint? There's no reason to spend all that money, work up all that mental sweat, and suffer the fear of failure if the place where you're trying to claw out a medical degree just isn't you. Some people like professors breathing down their necks: They think plastic pocket protectors are a fashion statement, and nothing makes them happier than tuition payments just slightly lower than the national debt. Maybe you're one of those people, and maybe you're not. This first chapter will help you find out for sure, and provide some guideposts to the academic institution that is right for you in terms of tuition, facilities, special programs, and peer groups.

• • • • • • • • • • • • • • • • • • •

"So we open the kid up, and what do you think we find? Three buttons, a thumb tack, and twenty-seven cents in change . . . . The parents couldn't afford to pay for the operation, so I kept the twenty-seven cents."
—Billy Wilder and I.A.I. Diamond
The Fortune Cookie, screenplay, 1966

Choosing a medical school should be exciting, never intimidating. You should be pumped and raring to go. With the help of this book, picking a school should feel like the exhilaration of extreme sports instead of just more homework. So hook yourself up and stand in the door. This is the jumping-off place—Geronimo!

"Pain is a more terrible lord of mankind than even death himself."
—Dr. Albert Schweitzer

LEAST EXPENSIVE TUITION

Bargain basement tuition is almost always available only at state colleges and universities, and, even then, is exclusively available for residents of the state. There is one medical school that is free, but not exactly without cost: You must wear the uniform of some branch of the U.S. Armed Forces to attend the Uniformed Services University of Health Sciences School of Medicine in Bethesda, Maryland. The schools in the following list charge in-state tuition under $7,000 per year.

University of North Carolina School of Medicine, Chapel Hill, NC	$2,430
Medical College of Georgia, Augusta, GA	$5,292
University of New Mexico School of Medicine, Albuquerque, NM	$5,331
University of Alabama School of Medicine, Birmingham, AL	$5,708
Baylor College of Medicine, Houston, TX	$6,550
Texas Tech University Health Sciences Center School of Medicine, Lubbock, TX	$6,550
University of Texas Medical School at Galveston, TX	$6,550
University of Texas Houston Medical School, Houston, TX	$6,550
University of Mississippi School of Medicine, Jackson, MS	$6,715

Louisiana State University School of Medicine, $6,774
New Orleans, LA

University of South Carolina School of Medicine, Columbia, SC $6,790

MOST EXPENSIVE TUITION

Here's some bad news. Not only must you have a pot of money to attend
these schools, but they also require that you have great grades, an outstanding record, solid references, and a high tolerance for rejection
(they get lots of applicants even at these prices). These schools charge
tuition exceeding $23,000 per year. Most of the state universities in this
list have much lower tuition prices for state residents. Out-of-state
tuition prices are marked with an asterisk. Schools that have outrageous
tuition for everyone are not marked at all.

University of Colorado School of Medicine, Denver, CO	$49,849 *
Southern Illinois University School of Medicine, Springfield, IL	$36,981 *
University of Illinois at Chicago College of Medicine, Chicago, IL	$32,780*
Boston University School of Medicine, Boston, MA	$31,520
Michigan State University College of Human Medicine, East Lansing, MI	$31,002 *
George Washington University School of Medicine and Health Sciences, Washington, DC	$30,200
Finch University of Health Sciences Chicago Medical School, Chicago, IL	$29,980
Oregon Health Sciences University School of Medicine, Portland, OR	$29,756 *
University of Minnesota Medical School, Minneapolis, MN	$29,112 *
University of Minnesota School of Medicine, Duluth, MN	$29,112 *
Tufts University School of Medicine, Boston, MA	$28,800

Ohio State University College of Medicine, Columbus, OH	$28,305
University of Vermont College of Medicine, Burlington, VT	$27,850 *
University of Southern California School of Medicine, Los Angeles, CA	$27,820
Washington University School of Medicine, St. Louis, MO	$27,435
Loyola University, Stritch School of Medicine, Chicago, IL	$27,150
Albany Medical College, Albany, NY	$26,613 *
Tulane University School of Medicine, New Orleans, LA	$26,610
Northwestern University Medical School, Chicago, IL	$26,592
University of Missouri School of Medicine, Columbia, MO	$26,579 *
Temple University School of Medicine, Philadelphia, PA	$26,286 *
New York Medical College, Valhalla, NY	$26,150
University of Pennsylvania School of Medicine, Philadelphia, PA	$25,880
St. Louis University School of Medicine, St. Louis, MO	$25,600
University of Michigan Medical School, Ann Arbor, MI	$25,514
Yeshiva University, Albert Einstein College of Medicine, Bronx, NY	$25,450
Stanford University School of Medicine, Stanford, CA	$25,350
Thomas Jefferson University, Jefferson Medical College, Philadelphia, PA	$25,235
Columbia University School of Medicine, New York, NY	$25,164
Brown University School of Medicine, Providence, RI	$24,984
Yale University School of Medicine, New Haven, CT	$24,700
Duke University School of Medicine, Durham, NC	$24,650
Case Western University School of Medicine, Cleveland, OH	$24,500
Creighton University School of Medicine, Omaha, NE	$24,254
University of Miami School of Medicine, Miami, FL	$24,190
Harvard Medical School, Cambridge, MA	$24,150

Medical College of Hampton Roads, Eastern Virginia Medical School, Norfolk, VA	$24,000
Medical College of Wisconsin, Milwaukee, WI	$23,909
Rush University Medical College, Chicago, IL	$23,868
University of Rochester School of Medicine and Dentistry, Rochester, NY	$23,800
University of Iowa College of Medicine, Iowa City, IA	$23,360
University of Pittsburgh School of Medicine, Pittsburgh, PA	$23,270
Dartmouth College Medical School, Hanover, NH	$23,260
Wake Forest University, Bowman Gray School of Medicine, Winston–Salem, NC	$23,000

HIGHEST FEES

While we're talking money, you should be aware that many schools charge a fee for services, equipment (microscopes, for example), facilities (labs, et cetera), and other miscellaneous charges in addition to your tuition. Your parents hocked the farm, the loans are in place, and you think you're ready for class, but . . . don't forget those pesky fees. For instance, although the University of California School of Medicine at San Diego has zero tuition for in-state students, they have the highest fees in the nation at $10,617. What's worse, many of the schools on the following list have the temerity to charge huge tuition and still bump up the fees into thousands of dollars.

University of California School of Medicine, San Diego, CA	$9,287
UCLA School of Medicine, Los Angeles, CA	$9,258
University of California School of Medicine, Davis, CA	$8,922
University of California School of Medicine, San Francisco, CA	$8,753
Dartmouth Medical School, Hanover, NH	$3,900
New York University School of Medicine, New York, NY	$3,810
University of Alabama School of Medicine, Birmingham, AL	$2,663

Oregon Health Sciences University School of Medicine, Portland, OR	$2,139
Meharry Medical College, Nashville, TN	$2,000
Morehouse College School of Medicine, Atlanta, GA	$1,986
Johns Hopkins University School of Medicine, Baltimore, MD	$1,910
University of Nevada School of Medicine, Reno, NV	$1,894
University of South Dakota School of Medicine, Vermillion, SD	$1,891
University of Colorado School of Medicine, Denver, CO	$1,805
Columbia University School of Physicians and Surgeons, New York, NY	$1,637
Rush Medical College of Rush University, Chicago, IL	$1,600
Baylor College of Medicine, Houston, TX	$1,559
Harvard Medical School, Cambridge. MA	$1,559

HIGHEST MCAT SCORES

The MCAT is a test of verbal reasoning, writing ability, and knowledge of physical and biological sciences. Your MCAT score is a prime factor in your application. The following list shows the schools that could be considered the toughest schools to get into because they require an average overall MCAT score of 10 or higher. Note that some very competitive schools, such as Johns Hopkins University School of Medicine, do not require the MCAT at all.

University of California School of Medicine, San Diego, CA	12
Washington University School of Medicine, St. Louis, MO	11.4
Cornell University Medical School, New York, NY	11
Harvard Medical School, Cambridge, MA	11
University of California School of Medicine, San Francisco, CA	11
Stanford University School of Medicine, Stanford, CA	10.9
Vanderbilt University School of Medicine, Nashville, TN	10.8

University of Chicago, Pritzker School of Medicine, Chicago, IL	10.6
University of Michigan Medical School, Ann Arbor, MI	10.5
University of Pennsylvania School of Medicine, Philadelphia, PA	10.5
University of Pittsburgh School of Medicine, Pittsburgh, PA	10.5
University of Utah School of Medicine, Salt Lake City, UT	10.5
Creighton University School of Medicine, Omaha, NE	10.4
University of Washington School of Medicine, Seattle, WA	10.2
Mayo Medical School, Rochester, MN	10.1
University of Texas Southwestern Medical Center, Dallas, TX	10.1
University of California School of Medicine, Davis, CA	10.1
University of Massachusetts Medical School, Worcester, MA	10.1
Yeshiva University, Albert Einstein School of Medicine, Bronx, NY	10
Baylor College of Medicine, Houston, TX	10
Columbia University College of Physicians and Surgeons. New York, NY	10
George Washington University School of Medicine and Health Sciences, Washington, DC	10
Georgetown University School of Medicine, Washington, DC	10
New York University School of Medicine, New York, NY	10
Oregon Health Sciences University School of Medicine, Portland, OR	10
SUNY at Stony Brook School of Medicine Health Sciences Center, Stony Brook, NY	10
Tulane University School of Medicine, New Orleans, LA	10
University of California College of Medicine, Irvine, CA	10
University of Illinois College of Medicine, Chicago, IL	10
University of Minnesota Medical School, Minneapolis, MN	10
University of Southern California School of Medicine, Los Angeles, CA	10
University of Virginia School of Medicine, Charlottesville, VA	10

FOR THOSE WHO CAN'T TAKE REJECTION

Schools with High Acceptance Rates

Nobody likes to be turned down. Rejection kicks in when you reach the age of 13, and then it never stops. If you can't stand being told to take a hike, consider attending a school with a record of accepting a high percentage of the people who apply. Don't give up just yet: Try the schools petitioned by fewer applicants, who are thereby more likely to let you in. Note that many of these schools heavily favor in-state applicants (and might even actively discourage out-of-state applicants), which can account for their relatively low number of applicants.

	Applications	Acceptances
Medical College of Georgia School of Medicine, Augusta	1,786	257
SUNY Buffalo	3,786	460
Texas A&M College of Medicine, College Station, TX	1,577	200
Texas Tech University Medical School, Lubbock, TX	1,697	314
University of Alabama–Birmingham, School of Medicine	2,106	238
University of Arkansas College of Medicine, Little Rock, AR	890	151
University of Kansas School of Medicine, Kansas City, KS	1,936	210
University of Massachusetts Medical School, Worcester, MA	1,051	150
University of Minnesota School of Medicine, Minneapolis, MN	2,330	258
University of Mississippi School of Medicine, Jackson, MS	630	122

University of Missouri School of Medicine, Columbia, MO	1,123	125
University of North Dakota School of Medicine and Health Sciences, Grand Forks, ND	370	82
University of Oklahoma School of Medicine, Oklahoma City, OK	1,126	151
University of Tennessee College of Medicine, Memphis, TN	1,959	258
University of Texas Southwestern Medical Center, Dallas, TX	3,418	376

FOR SNOB APPEAL

Schools with Low Acceptance Rates

So you've got great grades, a good record, outstanding references, and will get into just about any law school you want to attend? Then pick a school that's picky. Exclusivity can be a good thing as long as you're not part of the crowd being excluded. The Marine Corps does it: "We're looking for a few good men." Go for the snob appeal. These schools accept 20 percent or less of the students who apply to them.

	Applications	Acceptances
Boston University School of Medicine, Boston, MA	11,586	149
Brown University School of Medicine Providence, RI	2,329	135
Creighton University School of Medicine, Omaha, NE	7,735	176
Dartmouth Medical School, Hanover, NH	7,898	226
Duke University School of Medicine, Durham, NC	7,181	210
Eastern Virginia Medical School, Norfolk, VA	7,278	223

Emory University School of Medicine, Atlanta, GA	8,612	114
Finch University of Health Sciences, Chicago, IL	12,798	166
Georgetown University School of Medicine, Washington, DC	10,984	309
Loyola University, Stritch School of Medicine, Chicago, IL	10,106	312
Mayo Medical School, Rochester, MN	3,900	90
Stanford Medical School, Stanford, CA	6,724	234
Jefferson Medical College, Philadelphia, PA	11,189	340
Tulane University School of Medicine, New Orleans, LA	10,782	304
University of Southern California School of Medicine, Los Angeles	6,488	150
Wake Forest University, Bowman Gray School of Medicine	7,884	210
University of Medicine and Dentistry of New Jersey, Piscataway	3,973	356
Yeshiva University, Albert Einstein School of Medicine, NY	9,135	180

ANONYMITY IS THE BEST DEFENSE

Schools with Large Enrollments

Although most med schools have a student population of 600–800 students, there are some larger schools out there. This doesn't mean that you'll be able to hide in a crowd—med schools are still relatively small places, and after four years you'll know your classmates pretty well. If you're an extrovert who thrives on a constant parade of people and personalities, these larger schools might be for you.

University of Illinois Chicago College of Medicine, Chicago, IL	1,321
Indiana University School of Medicine, Indianapolis, IN	1,103
Philadelphia University of Osteopathic Medicine, Philadelphia, PA	1,093
Wayne State University School of Medicine, Detroit, MI	1,049
Thomas Jefferson University Medical College, Philadelphia, PA	902
University of Minnesota School of Medicine, Minneapolis, MN	887
Ohio State University College of Medicine, Columbus, OH	844
University of Texas Houston Medical School, Houston, TX	831
University of Texas Southwestern Medical Center, Dallas, TX	830
New York College of Osteopathic Medicine, Old Westbury, NY	827
University of Texas Medical School of San Antonio, TX	826
University of Texas School of Medicine, Galveston, TX	820
SUNY Health Science Center Brooklyn Medical School, NY	812
University of Osteopathic Medicine and Health Sciences, Des Moines, IA	812
Medical College of Wisconsin, Milwaukee, WI	807

BIG FISH/SMALL POND
Schools with Small Enrollments

Do you like to stand out in a crowd? Would you flourish in a more intimate environment with a few well-chosen colleagues, a handpicked peer group of—let's say—325 people or fewer? The following schools have the smallest enrollments. Cadavers might outnumber students here. If you prefer a setting in which you'll know your fellow students really well, these smaller medical schools might be for you.

School	Enrollment
Midwestern College of Osteopathic Medicine, Glendale, AZ	103
University of Minnesota School of Medicine, Duluth, MN	110
University of Nebraska College of Medicine, Omaha, NE	123
Morehouse College School of Medicine, Atlanta, GA	152
Mayo Medical School, Rochester, MN	179
Marshall University School of Medicine, Huntington, WV	199
Mercer University School of Medicine, Macon, GA	206
University of Nevada School of Medicine, Reno, NV	208
Texas A&M University College of Medicine, College Station, TX	226
University of Hawaii, John A. Burns School of Medicine, Honolulu, HI	229
University of North Dakota School of Medicine, Grand Forks, ND	235
University of Southern Alabama School of Medicine, Mobile, AL	261
West Virginia School of Osteopathic Medicine, Lewisburg, WV	261
University of New England School of Osteopathic Medicine, Biddeford, ME	281
University of South Carolina School of Medicine, Columbia, SC	285
Southern Illinois University School of Medicine, Springfield, IL	290
University of Medicine and Dentistry of New Jersey, Newark, NJ	290
East Carolina University School of Medicine, Greenville, NC	302
Dartmouth Medical School, Hanover, NH	317

SPECIALIZING IN PRIMARY CARE

State-run schools form the mainstay of colleges emphasizing primary care. These schools accept state residents with extreme prejudice over out-of-staters, and offer low tuition with the hope that graduates will stick around and provide medical care to state residents. Some schools have "community service" requirements or absolve student loans in exchange for two years of state service. Some schools with religious affiliations also emphasize primary care for the "medically underserved," as do certain "comprehensive" medical institutions, such as Mayo Medical School, which is distinguished as a research and primary care college. Here are some schools specializing in primary care.

East Carolina State University School of Medicine, Greenville, NC

East Tennessee State University College of Medicine, Johnson City, TN

Medical College of Hampton Roads, Eastern Virginia Medical School, Norfolk, VA

George Washington University School of Medicine, Washington, DC

Loma Linda University School of Medicine, Loma Linda, CA

Louisiana State University School of Medicine, New Orleans, LA

Loyola University, Stritch School of Medicine, Chicago, IL

Mayo Medical School, Rochester, MN

Marshall University School of Medicine, Huntington, WV

Medical College of Ohio, Toledo, OH

Mercer University School of Medicine, Macon, GA

Michigan State University College of Human Medicine, East Lansing, MI

Morehouse College School of Medicine, Atlanta, GA

Northeastern Ohio University School of Medicine, Rootstown, OH

Southern Illinois University School of Medicine, Springfield, IL

Texas A&M University College of Medicine, College Station, TX

Texas Tech University School of Medicine, Lubbock, TX

University of Arkansas School of Medicine, Little Rock, AR

University of California College of Medicine, Irvine, CA

University of Connecticut School of Medicine, Farmington, CT

University of Iowa College of Medicine, Iowa City, IA

University of Kansas School of Medicine, Kansas City, KS

University of Louisville School of Medicine, Louisville, KY

University of Massachusetts Medical School, Worcester, MA

University of Minnesota School of Medicine, Duluth, MN

University of Mississippi School of Medicine, Jackson, MS

University of Missouri School of Medicine, Columbia, MO

University of Nebraska College of Medicine, Omaha, NE

University of North Dakota School of Medicine, Grand Forks, ND

University of Oklahoma School of Medicine, Oklahoma City, OK

University of South Alabama College of Medicine, Mobile, AL

University of South Carolina School of Medicine, Columbia, SC

University of South Dakota School of Medicine, Vermillion, SD

University of Tennessee College of Medicine, Memphis, TN

University of Vermont College of Medicine, Burlington, VT

University of Washington School of Medicine, Seattle, WA

Wright State University School of Medicine, Dayton, OH

DOCTOR AS MAD SCIENTIST

The Best Schools for Research

Someone had to invent the polio vaccine and birth control pills, and some of you will have to do research to tackle tomorrow's challenges as well. The best place to work on medical research is at one of the 62 members of the Association of American Universities, a prestigious affiliation of the leading research institutions in the United States and Canada. Here is a list of member institutions.

Brown University School of Medicine, Hanover, NH

Case Western Reserve University School of Medicine, Cleveland, OH

Columbia University School of Physicians and Surgeons, New York, NY

Cornell University Medical College, New York, NY

Duke University School of Medicine, Durham, NC

Emory University School of Medicine, Atlanta, GA

Harvard Medical School, Cambridge, MA

Indiana University School of Medicine, Indianapolis, IN

Johns Hopkins University School of Medicine, Baltimore, MD

Michigan State University College of Human Medicine,
East Lansing, MI

New York University School of Medicine, New York, NY

Northwestern University Medical School, Chicago, IL

Ohio State University College of Medicine, Columbus, OH

Pennsylvania State University School of Medicine, Hershey, PA

Stanford University School of Medicine, Stanford, CA

Tulane University School of Medicine, New Orleans, LA

University of Arizona College of Medicine, Tucson, AZ

University of California School of Medicine, Davis, CA

University of California College of Medicine, Irvine, CA

University of California School of Medicine, San Diego, CA

University of Chicago, Pritzker School of Medicine, Chicago, IL

University of Florida College of Medicine, Gainesville, FL

University of Kansas School of Medicine, Kansas City, KS

University of Michigan Medical School, Ann Arbor, MI

University of Minnesota School of Medicine, Minneapolis, MN

University of Missouri School of Medicine, Columbia, MO

University of North Carolina School of Medicine, Chapel Hill, NC

University of Pennsylvania School of Medicine, Philadelphia, PA

University of Pittsburgh School of Medicine, Pittsburgh, PA

University of Rochester School of Medicine and Dentistry, Rochester, NY

University of Southern California School of Medicine, Los Angeles, CA

University of Virginia School of Medicine, Charlottesville, VA

University of Washington School of Medicine, Seattle, WA

University of Wisconsin School of Medicine, Madison, WI

Vanderbilt University School of Medicine, Nashville, TN

Washington University School of Medicine, St. Louis, MO

Yale University School of Medicine, New Haven, CT

KNOCK 'EM OUT

Schools with Specialties in Anesthesiology

Ancient Egyptians are known to have used surgery thousands of years ago, but anesthesiology always lagged behind—patients were once put out with a sharp mallet blow to the head (People in pain are so much easier to deal with when they're asleep, don't you think?). Anesthesiology is the medical study of administering anesthetics before and during surgery and other medical procedures, so the patient feels no pain. But leave your hammer home these days, because there's a lot more to it than knowing how to mix a good Harvey Wallbanger. If you're interested in anesthesiology as a specialty, here's a state-by-state list of the schools for you.

Alabama

University of Alabama School of Medicine

University of South Alabama College of Medicine

Arkansas

University of Arkansas, College of Medicine

California

University of California School of Medicine, Davis

University of California College of Medicine, Irvine

UCLA School of Medicine, Los Angeles

University of Southern California School of Medicine, Los Angeles

Loma Linda University School of Medicine, Loma Linda

University of California School of Medicine, San Diego

University of California School of Medicine, San Francisco

Colorado

University of Colorado School of Medicine

Connecticut

University of Connecticut School of Medicine

Yale University School of Medicine

District of Columbia

George Washington University School of Medicine and Health Sciences

Georgetown University School of Medicine

Howard University College of Medicine

Florida

University of Florida College of Medicine

University of South Florida College of Medicine

Georgia

Emory University School of Medicine

Medical College of Georgia

Illinois

Northwestern University School of Medicne

University of Chicago, Pritzker School of Medicine

University of Illinois College of Medicine

Loyola University, Stritch School of Medicine

Indiana

Indiana University School of Medicine

Iowa

University of Iowa College of Medicine

Kansas

University of Kansas School of Medicine

Kentucky

University of Kentucky College of Medicine

University of Louisville School of Medicine

Louisiana

Louisiana State University School of Medicine, New Orleans

Tulane University School of Medicine

Louisiana State University School of Medicine, Shreveport

Maryland

Johns Hopkins University School of Medicine

University of Maryland School of Medicine

Massachusetts

Boston University School of Medicine

University of Massachusetts School of Medicine

Michigan

University of Michigan Medical School

Minnesota

University of Minnesota Medical School, Minneapolis

Mayo Medical School

Mississippi

University of Mississippi School of Medicine

Missouri

University of Missouri School of Medicine

St. Louis University School of Medicine

Nebraska

University of Nebraska College of Medicine

New Hampshire

Dartmouth Medical School

New Jersey

University of Medicine and Dentistry of New Jersey, Newark

University of Medicine and Dentistry of New Jersey, Piscataway

New Mexico

University of New Mexico School of Medicine

New York

SUNY Health Science Center School of Medicine, Brooklyn

SUNY at Buffalo School of Medicine and Biomedical Sciences

New York University School of Medicine

University of Rochester School of Medicine and Dentistry

SUNY Stony Brook School of Medicine Health Sciences Center

New York Medical College

North Carolina

University of North Carolina School of Medicine, Chapel Hill

Duke University School of Medicine

Ohio

University of Cincinnati School of Medicine

Ohio State University School of Medicine

Medical College of Ohio

Oregon

Oregon Health Sciences University School of Medicine

Pennsylvania

Thomas Jefferson University, Jefferson Medical College

Medical College of Pennsylvania and Hahnemann University School of Medicine

University of Pennsylvania School of Medicine

Temple University School of Medicine

Pennsylvania State University College of Medicine, Hershey

University of Pittsburgh School of Medicine

South Carolina

Medical University of South Carolina College of Medicine

Tennessee

University of Tennessee College of Medicine

Vanderbilt University School of Medicine

Texas

Baylor College of Medicine

University of Texas Houston Medical School

University of Texas Medical School at Galveston

Texas A&M University Health Science Center

Texas Tech University Health Science Center School of Medicine, Lubbock

University of Texas Southwestern Medical Center at Dallas

University of Texas Medical School at San Antonio

Utah

University of Utah School of Medicine

Virginia

University of Virginia School of Medicine

Viringia Commonwealth University, Medical College of Virginia

Washington

University of Washington School of Medicine

West Virginia

West Virginia University School of Medicine

Wisconsin

University of Wisconsin School of Medicine

Medical College of Wisconsin

NUCLEAR WAR ON DISEASE

Schools Excelling in Nuclear Medicine

No, it has nothing to do with A-bombs or magic bullets: Nuclear medicine uses nuclear isotopes in techniques that allow physicians to see and understand organs deep within the body. Radionuclides, unstable atoms that emit radiation spontaneously, are used to diagnose and treat diseases. If you like wearing yellow rubber clothes, love things that glow in the dark, and don't mind a little radiation exposure now and then, the nukes may be for you. Here are some schools that excel in nuclear medicine.

Oregon Health Sciences University School of Medicine, Portland, OR

St. Louis University School of Medicine, St. Louis, MO

SUNY at Buffalo School of Medicine and Biomedical Sciences

University of Iowa School of Medicine, Iowa City, IA

University of Nebraska College of Medicine, Omaha, NE

University of Tennessee College of Medicine, Memphis

University of Washington School of Medicine, Seattle, WA

OB-GYN

If you're reading this, you can probably thank your mother's OB-GYN. Most likely, that doctor was heavily responsible for successfully bringing you into the world. So, if you think you might be interested in helping future mommies bring their babies safely into the world, specializing in OB-GYN might be for you. Here are a list of several schools that offer programs in obstetrics and gynecology.

Alabama

University of Alabama School of Medicine

University of South Alabama College of Medicine

Arizona

University of Arizona College of Medicine

Arkansas

University of Arkansas, Medical Sciences College of Medicine

California

University of California School of Medicine, Davis

University of California College of Medicine, Irvine

UCLA School of Medicine

University of Southern California School of Medicine

Loma Linda University School of Medicine

University of California School of Medicine, San Diego

University of California School of Medicine, San Francisco

Stanford University School of Medicine

Colorado

University of Colorado School of Medicine

Connecticut

University of Connecticut School of Medicine

Yale University School of Medicine

District of Columbia

Georgetown University School of Medicine

George Washington University School of Medicine and Health Sciences

Florida

University of Florida College of Medicine

University of South Florida College of Medicine

Georgia

Emory University School of Medicine

Medical College of Georgia

Hawaii

University of Hawaii, John A. Burrs School of Medicine

Illinois

Northwestern University School of Medicine

University of Chicago, Pritzker School of Medicine

University of Illinois College of Medicine

Loyola University, Stritch School of Medicine

Southern Illinois School of Medicine

Indiana

Indiana University School of Medicine

Iowa

University of Iowa Hospitals School of Medicine

Kansas

University of Kansas School of Medicine

Kentucky

University of Kentucky College of Medicine

University of Louisville School of Medicine

Louisiana

Louisiana State University School of Medicine, Shreveport

Tulane University School of Medicine

Louisiana State University School of Medicine, New Orleans

Maryland

Johns Hopkins University School of Medicine

University of Maryland School of Medicine

Massachusetts

University of Massachusetts School of Medicine

Michigan

University of Michigan Medical School

Wayne State University School of Medicine

Minnesota

University of Minnesota School of Medicine

Mayo Medical School

Mississippi

University of Mississippi School of Medicine

Missouri

University of Missouri School of Medicine

St. Louis University School of Medicine

Nebraska

University of Nebraska College of Medicine

Creighton University School of Medicine

Nevada

University of Nevada School of Medicine

New Jersey

University of Medicine and Dentistry of New Jersey, Newark

University of Medicine and Dentistry of New Jersey, Piscataway

New Mexico

University of New Mexico School of Medicine

New York

New York University School of Medicine

SUNY Health Science Center at Brooklyn College of Medicine

University of Rochester School of Medicine and Dentistry

SUNY at Buffalo School of Medicine and Biomedical Sciences

SUNY Health Science Center at Syracuse College of Medicine

North Carolina

University of North Carolina School of Medicine, Chapel Hill

Duke University School of Medicine

East Carolina University School of Medicine

Ohio

University of Cincinnati College of Medicine

Medical College of Ohio, Toledo

Northeastern Ohio Universities College of Medicine, Rootsville

Ohio State University College of Medicine, Columbus

Wright State University School of Medicine, Dayton

Oklahoma

University of Oklahoma College of Medicine

Oregon

Oregon Health Sciences University School of Medicine

Pennsylvania

Thomas Jefferson University, Jefferson Medical College

Medical College of Pennsylvania and Hahnemann University School of Medicine

University of Pennsylvania School of Medicine

Temple University School of Medicine

Pennsylvania State University College of Medicine

University of Pittsburgh School of Medicine

South Carolina

Medical University of South Carolina College of Medicine

Tennessee

University of Tennessee College of Medicine

East Tennessee State University College of Medicine

Vanderbilt University School of Medicine

Texas

Baylor College of Medicine

University of Texas, Houston Medical School

University of Texas Medical School at Galveston

Texas A&M University Health Science Center, College Station

Texas Tech University Health Science Center School of Medicine, Lubbock

University of Texas, Southwestern Medical Center at Dallas

Utah

University of Utah School of Medicine

Virginia

University of Virginia School of Medicine

Virginia Commonwealth University Medical College of Virginia

Medical College of Hampton Roads, Eastern Virginia Medical School

Washington

University of Washington School of Medicine

West Virginia

West Virginia University School of Medicine

Marshall University School of Medicine

Wisconsin

University of Wisconsin School of Medicine

Medical College of Wisconsin

THE BONEYARD

Schools with Special Programs in Orthopedic Medicine

Only God can make a knee . . . or an elbow or a wrist for that matter. But there's plenty of work repairing joints and broken bones in this country. Extreme sports, skiing, bungee jumping, over-40 guys playing football at their high school reunions, all these things have combined to make orthopedics a growing specialty in the United States And as the population steadily shifts to elderly, hip replacements are bound to increase. Grab this specialty and don't let go. The following state-by-state list contains schools with special programs in orthopedic medicine and surgery.

Alabama

University of South Alabama College of Medicine

Arizona

University of Arizona College of Medicine

Arkansas

University of Arkansas For Medical Sciences College of Medicine

California

University of California School of Medicine, Davis

University of California College of Medicine, Irvine

UCLA School of Medicine

University of Southern California School of Medicine

Loma Linda University School of Medicine

University of California School of Medicine, San Diego

University of California School of Medicine, San Francisco

Stanford University School of Medicine

Colorado

University of Colorado School of Medicine

Connecticut

University of Connecticut School of Medicine

Yale University School of Medicine

District of Columbia

Georgetown University School of Medicine

George Washington University School of Medicine and Health Sciences

Howard University College of Medicine

Florida

University of Florida College of Medicine

Georgia

Emory University School of Medicine

Medical College of Georgia

Hawaii

University of Hawaii, John A. Burrs School of Medicine

Illinois

Northwestern University School of Medicine

University of Chicago, Pritzker School of Medicine

University of Illinois College of Medicine

Loyola University, Stritch School of Medicine

Southern Illinois School of Medicine

Indiana

Indiana University School of Medicine

Iowa

University of Iowa Hospitals School of Medicine

Kansas

University of Kansas School of Medicine

Kentucky

University of Kentucky College of Medicine

University of Louisville School of Medicine

Louisiana

Louisiana State University School of Medicine, Shreveport

Tulane University School of Medicine

Louisiana State University School of Medicine, New Orleans

Maryland

Johns Hopkins University School of Medicine

University of Maryland School of Medicine

Massachusetts

Boston University School of Medicine

Harvard Medical School

University of Massachusetts School of Medicine

Michigan

Michigan State University College of Human Medicine

University of Michigan Medical School

Wayne State University School of Medicine

Minnesota

University of Minnesota School of Medicine

Mayo Medical School

Mississippi

University of Mississippi School of Medicine

Missouri

University of Missouri School of Medicine

St. Louis University School of Medicine

Nebraska

Creighton University School of Medicine

New Hampshire

Dartmouth Medical School

New Jersey

University of Medicine and Dentistry of New Jersey, Newark

University of Medicine and Dentistry of New Jersey, Piscataway

New Mexico

University of New Mexico School of Medicine

New York

New York University School of Medicine

SUNY Health Science Center at Brooklyn College of Medicine

University of Rochester School of Medicine and Dentistry

SUNY at Buffalo School of Medicine and Biomedical Sciences

SUNY Health Science Center at Syracuse College of Medicine

North Carolina

University of North Carolina School of Medicine, Chapel Hill

Duke University School of Medicine

Ohio

University of Cincinnati College of Medicine

Medical College of Ohio, Toledo

Northeastern Ohio Universities College of Medicine, Rootsville

Ohio State University College of Medicine, Columbus

Wright State University School of Medicine, Dayton

Oklahoma

University of Oklahoma College of Medicine

Oregon

Oregon Health Sciences University School of Medicine

Pennsylvania

Thomas Jefferson University, Jefferson Medical College

Medical College of Pennsylvania and Hahnemann University
School of Medicine

University of Pennsylvania School of Medicine

Temple University School of Medicine

Pennsylvania State University College of Medicine

University of Pittsburgh School of Medicine

South Carolina

Medical University of South Carolina College of Medicine

Tennessee

University of Tennessee College of Medicine

Vanderbilt University School of Medicine

Texas

University of Texas Houston Medical School

University of Texas Medical School at Galveston

Texas A&M University Health Science Center, College Station

Texas Tech University Health Science Center School of Medicine, Lubbock

University of Texas Southwestern Medical Center at Dallas

Utah

University of Utah School of Medicine

Virginia

University of Virginia School of Medicine

Virginia Commonwealth University Medical College of Virginia

Washington

University of Washington School of Medicine

West Virginia

West Virginia University School of Medicine

Marshall University School of Medicine

Wisconsin

University of Wisconsin School of Medicine

Medical College of Wisconsin

PLASTIC SURGERY

Plastic surgeons' main concern is to correct disfigurements of the face or body caused by injury, disease, or birth defects. However, much of their time is spent correcting less serious birth defects like large proboscises, lips that aren't sufficiently pouty, liposuctioning out some of that subcutaneous fat laid on a few decades after the patient was born, and snipping and tucking away at those birth defects called wrinkles that show up about 50 years after most people are brought into the world. Here are some schools with programs in plastic surgery.

Johns Hopkins University School of Medicine, Baltimore, MD

Loma Linda University School of Medicine, Loma Linda, CA

Medical College of Wisconsin, Milwaukee, WI

Northwestern University Medical School, Chicago, IL

Ohio State University College of Medicine, Columbus, OH

St. Louis University School of Medicine, St. Louis, MO

Southern Illinois University School of Medicine, Springfield, IL

Stanford University School of Medicine, Stanford, CA

University of Chicago, Pritzker School of Medicine, Chicago, IL

University of Cincinnati College of Medicine, Cincinnati, OH

University of Kentucky College of Medicine, Lexington, KY

University of Michigan Medical School, Ann Arbor, MI

University of Missouri School of Medicine, Columbia, MO

University of Pennsylvania School of Medicine, Philadelphia, PA

University of Pittsburgh School of Medicine, Pittsburgh, PA

University of Rochester School of Medicine and Dentistry, Rochester, NY

University of South Florida College of Medicine, Tampa, FL

University of Texas Southwestern Medical School, Dallas, TX

University of Washington School of Medicine, Seattle, WA

PSYCHIATRY

To become a psychiatrist, you have to spend almost twice as long in school as the normal doctor, and it's going to cost you an arm and a leg more than the arm and a leg you've already spent. But look at the bright side: Your patients may talk your ears off, but they won't be coughing in your face or barfing on your shoes . . . usually. If this specialty is for you, pick a school from the following state-by-state list of medical schools with special programs leading to certification as a psychiatrist.

Alabama

University of Alabama School of Medicine

University of South Alabama College of Medicine

Arizona

University of Arizona College of Medicine

Arkansas

University of Arkansas for Medical Sciences College of Medicine

California

University of California School of Medicine, Davis

University of California College of Medicine, Irvine

UCLA School of Medicine

University of Southern California School of Medicine

Loma Linda University School of Medicine

University of California School of Medicine, San Diego

University of California School of Medicine, San Francisco

Stanford University School of Medicine

Colorado

University of Colorado School of Medicine

Connecticut

University of Connecticut School of Medicine

Yale University School of Medicine

District of Columbia

Georgetown University School of Medicine

George Washington University School of Medicine and Health Sciences

Howard University College of Medicine

Florida

University of Florida College of Medicine

University of South Florida College of Medicine

Georgia

Emory University School of Medicine

Medical College of Georgia

Morehouse College School of Medicine

Hawaii

University of Hawaii, John A. Burrs School of Medicine

Illinois

Northwestern University School of Medicine

University of Chicago, Pritzker School of Medicine

University of Illinois College of Medicine

Loyola University, Stritch School of Medicine

Southern Illinois School of Medicine

Finch University of Health Sciences Chicago Medical School

Indiana

Indiana University School of Medicine

Iowa

University of Iowa Hospitals School of Medicine

Kansas

University of Kansas School of Medicine

Kentucky

University of Kentucky College of Medicine

University of Louisville School of Medicine

Louisiana

Tulane University School of Medicine

Louisiana State University School of Medicine, New Orleans

Maryland

Johns Hopkins University School of Medicine

University of Maryland School of Medicine

Massachusetts

Boston University School of Medicine

Harvard Medical School

University of Massachusetts School of Medicine

Michigan

Michigan State University College of Human Medicine

University of Michigan Medical School

Wayne State University School of Medicine

Minnesota

University of Minnesota School of Medicine

Mayo Medical School

Mississippi

University of Mississippi School of Medicine

Missouri

University of Missouri School of Medicine

St. Louis University School of Medicine

Nebraska

University of Nebraska School of Medicine

Creighton University School of Medicine

New Hampshire

Dartmouth Medical School

New Jersey

University of Medicine and Dentistry of New Jersey, Newark

University of Medicine and Dentistry of New Jersey, Piscataway

New Mexico

University of New Mexico School of Medicine

New York

New York University School of Medicine

Mt. Sinai School of Medicine

Cornell University School of Medicine

New York Medical College

SUNY Health Science Center at Brooklyn College of Medicine

University of Rochester School of Medicine and Dentistry

SUNY at Buffalo School of Medicine and Biomedical Sciences

SUNY Health Science Center at Syracuse College of Medicine

North Carolina

University of North Carolina School of Medicine, Chapel Hill

Duke University School of Medicine

East Carolina University School of Medicine

North Dakota

University of North Dakota School of Medicine

Ohio

University of Cincinnati College of Medicine

Medical College of Ohio, Toledo

Northeastern Ohio Universities College of Medicine

Ohio State University College of Medicine

Wright State University School of Medicine

Oklahoma

University of Oklahoma College of Medicine

Oregon

Oregon Health Sciences University School of Medicine

Pennsylvania

Thomas Jefferson University, Jefferson Medical College

Medical College of Pennsylvania and Hahnemann University School of Medicine

University of Pennsylvania School of Medicine

Temple University School of Medicine

Pennsylvania State University College of Medicine

University of Pittsburgh School of Medicine

Rhode Island

Brown University School of Medicine

South Carolina

Medical University of South Carolina College of Medicine

South Dakota

University of South Dakota School of Medicine

Tennessee

East Tennessee University School of Medicine

Meharry Medical College School of Medicine

University of Tennessee College of Medicine

Vanderbilt University School of Medicine

Texas

University of Texas Houston Medical School

University of Texas Medical School at Galveston

Texas A&M University Health Science Center, College Station

Texas Tech University Health Science Center School of Medicine, Lubbock

University of Texas Southwestern Medical Center at Dallas

Utah

University of Utah School of Medicine

Virginia

University of Virginia School of Medicine

Virginia Commonwealth University Medical College of Virginia

Medical College of Hampton Roads, Eastern Virginia Medical School

Washington

University of Washington School of Medicine

West Virginia

West Virginia University School of Medicine

Marshall University School of Medicine

Wisconsin

University of Wisconsin School of Medicine

Medical College of Wisconsin

KID DOCS

Schools with Pediatric Programs

As any parent can tell you—ask your own—kids are just little satchels of germs running around trying to infect each other. Failing that, they will throw themselves off the nearest chair, housetop, or swing set in order to break a limb or gash themselves badly enough to need stitches. Children prove that we are all projectile vomiters—we just learn with age to aim down.

There are two major requirements to keep in mind: You have to love children, and you have to be agile enough to catch that kid who doesn't want a shot before he makes it out the front door of your office. The job has its rewards—kids do say things that will keep you laughing, and there's nothing worth more than the smile on the face of a four-year-old. Here is a state-by-state list of the medical schools with pediatric programs.

Alabama

University of Alabama School of Medicine

University of South Alabama College of Medicine

Arkansas

University of Arkansas for Medical Sciences College of Medicine

California

University of Southern California School of Medicine

Loma Linda University School of Medicine

University of California School of Medicine, San Diego

Florida

University of Florida College of Medicine

Hawaii

University of Hawaii, John A. Burrs School of Medicine

Illinois

University of Chicago, Pritzker School of Medicine

University of Illinois College of Medicine

Loyola University, Stritch School of Medicine

Southern Illinois School of Medicine

Indiana

Indiana University School of Medicine

Kansas

University of Kansas School of Medicine

Kentucky

University of Kentucky College of Medicine

University of Louisville School of Medicine

Louisiana

Louisiana State University School of Medicine, Shreveport

Louisiana State University School of Medicine, New Orleans

Maryland

University of Maryland School of Medicine

Michigan

Michigan State University College of Human Medicine

University of Michigan Medical School

Wayne State University School of Medicine

Minnesota

University of Minnesota School of Medicine

Mississippi

University of Mississippi School of Medicine

Missouri

University of Missouri School of Medicine

St. Louis University School of Medicine

Nebraska

Creighton University School of Medicine

New Jersey

University of Medicine and Dentistry of New Jersey, Newark

University of Medicine and Dentistry of New Jersey, Piscataway

New York

SUNY Health Science Center at Brooklyn College of Medicine

University of Rochester School of Medicine and Dentistry

SUNY at Buffalo School of Medicine and Biomedical Science

North Carolina

University of North Carolina School of Medicine, Chapel Hill

Duke University School of Medicine

East Carolina University School of Medicine

Ohio

University of Cincinnati College of Medicine

Medical College of Ohio, Toledo

Northeastern Ohio Universities College of Medicine

Ohio State University College of Medicine

Wright State University School of Medicine

Oklahoma

University of Oklahoma College of Medicine

Pennsylvania

Pennsylvania State University College of Medicine

Tennessee

University of Tennessee College of Medicine

Vanderbilt University School of Medicine

Texas

University of Texas Houston Medical School

University of Texas Medical School at Galveston

Texas A&M University Health Science Center, College Station

Texas Tech University Health Science Center School of Medicine, Lubbock

Utah

University of Utah School of Medicine

Virginia

Virginia Commonwealth University Medical College of Virginia

West Virginia

West Virginia University School of Medicine

Marshall University School of Medicine

Wisconsin

Medical College of Wisconsin

MANO A MANO

Schools with At Least Two Faculty Per Student

According to the figures they publish, some schools would appear to have a faculty in brigade or even division strength (Harvard: 7,591). This does not mean that each student is escorted from class to class by a phalanx of academics; or that lectures are conducted in quadrophonic sound with four teachers pontificating simultaneously. Rather, it means that some schools lump together just about every one who has anything to do with the medical school—part-time instructors, unpaid volunteers, professors emeritus and others—in with their count of full-time faculty. Still, a higher ratio of faculty to students is a quality to be valued as you decide on the right medical school for you. Here are the schools with a ratio of faculty to students of two to one or better:

	Students	Faculty
Medical College of Pennsylvania and Hahnemann University School of Medicine	650	1,300
Brown University School of Medicine	321	704
Case Western Reserve University School of Medicine	582	1,372
Columbia University College of Physicians and Surgeons	601	4,571
Dartmouth Medical College (full time)	317	757
Harvard Medical School	741	7,591
Mayo Medical School	179	1,720
Northeastern Ohio Universities College of Medicine	421	1,700
Northwestern University Medical School	697	2,424
Ohio State College of Medicine	844	1,712
Rush Medical College of Rush University	489	2,673
Texas A&M College of Medicine	226	501
Thomas Jefferson University, Jefferson Medical College	902	3,002

Uniformed Services University School of Medicine	673	3,478
University of Chicago, Pritzker School of Medicine	421	1,150
University of Medicine and Dentistry of New Jersey, Newark (including volunteers)	696	1,927
University of Medicine and Dentistry of New Jersey, Piscataway (including volunteers)	623	2,438
University of Michigan Medical School	653	1,754
University of Pennsylvania School of Medicine	684	2,621
University of Pittsburgh School of Medicine	560	1,400
University of Rochester School of Medicine and Dentistry	405	966
Vanderbilt University School of Medicine	412	976
Washington University School of Medicine, St. Louis	576	1,164
Wright State University School of Medicine	371	1,612
Yeshiva University, Albert Einstein School of Medicine	720	3,510

ESPECIALLY FOR BOOKWORMS

Schools with the Largest Libraries

You'll be hitting the books big time in medical school. Not only will you need a great repository of knowledge in which to do your research, but you'll be in competition for many of the same books with your fellow students. Worse, you'll be vying with a lot of other very determined people for a comfy seat, with a little privacy, near a window. So it makes sense that the larger the library, and the bigger the target area, the easier it will be to get your hands on the text you want and find a place to curl up with it. But be warned: Big doesn't always mean accessible or tailored to your needs. Some libraries are large but built on a collection of esoteric junk that the donor of the building insisted that the library house. State system universities always look good in the number-of-branches department, but remember that the libraries listed as branches are usually at other schools with an entire student body fighting over access to those books as well. The following list is of universities with the largest libraries. The first number reflects the quantity of books; the second number refers to professional journals and periodicals to which the library subscribes.

	Volumes	Periodicals
University of Chicago, Pritzker School of Medicine	982,000	7,040
University of Illinois College of Medicine	710,000	6,925
University of California School of Medicine San Francisco	615,000	8,845
Columbia University College of Physicians and Surgeons	472,000	4,035
University of Minnesota Medical School	417,000 combined total	
Yale University School of Medicine	372,000	2,563
Harvard Medical School	372,000 combined total	
Washington University School of Medicine	367,000	3,255
Johns Hopkins University School of Medicine	346,000	3,720
University of Southern California School of Medicine	315,000 combined total	
Stanford University School of Medicine	291,000	3,040
Mayo Medical School	288,000	3,440
SUNY at Buffalo School of Medicine	270,000	2,780
Northwestern University Medical School	261,000	2,680
University of North Carolina School of Medicine	261,000	4,860
University of Maryland School of Medicine	252,000	3,120
SUNY Brooklyn College of Medicine	258,000 combined total	

University of Texas School of Medicine, Galveston	252,000	3,055
SUNY Stony Brook School of Medicine	244,000	4,435
Southern Illinois School of Medicine	237,000	1,690
Medical University of South Carolina	227,000	3,170
University of Rochester School of Medicine and Dentistry	224,000 combined total	
University of Michigan Medical School	216,000	3,035
Dartmouth Medical School	212,000	3,055
Duke University School of Medicine	210,000	5,065
University of Iowa School of Medicine	206,000	2,000
University of Missouri School of Medicine	204,000	2,045
University of Florida College of Medicine	202,000 combined total	

LARGEST SINGLE GROUP OF GUINEA PIGS

Schools with the Largest Hospitals

An important factor in learning is the clinical training facility, or hospital, at your disposal. Besides the possibility that you may need to be hospitalized for exhaustion yourself, it will be advantageous to have your training take place in one large hospital. It makes the job easier. Many schools rely on hospitals spread across a county. Here are the schools that use the single largest hospitals, as deduced by the number of beds:

	Number of Beds
Mayo Medical School, Rochester, MN	2,250
University of Miami School of Medicine, Miami, FL	2,215
University of Southern California School of Medicine, Los Angeles, CA	2,160
Harvard Medical School, Cambridge, MA	2,100

Washington University School of Medicine, St. Louis, MO	1,900
Cornell Medical School, New York, NY	1,510
University of Maryland School of Medicine, Baltimore, MD	1,480
Mt. Sinai School of Medicine, New York, NY	1,375
Indiana University School of Medicine, Indianapolis, IN	1,364
University of Iowa School of Medicine, Iowa City, IA	1,135
Johns Hopkins University School of Medicine, Baltimore, MD	1,150
Virginia Commonwealth University Medical College, Richmond, VA	1,080
Duke University School of Medicine, Durham, NC	1,075
Louisiana State University School of Medicine, Shreveport, LA	1,065
Rush Medical College of Rush University, Chicago, IL	930
University of Michigan Medical School, Ann Arbor, MI	914
Wake Forest University, Bowman Gray School of Medicine, Winston-Salem, NC	830
University of Alabama School of Medicine, Birmingham, AL	830
University of Chicago, Pritzker School of Medicine, Chicago, IL	782
University of Rochester School of Medicine and Dentistry, Rochester, NY	745
Albany Medical College, Albany, NY	685
University of North Carolina School of Medicine, Chapel Hill, NC	685

ROLLING IN DOUGH

Schools with the Biggest Research Budgets

You wouldn't want the school of your choice to suddenly go belly-up in the middle of your studies, despite the thousands of dollars you were pouring into its coffers. So it might be best to pick a medical school that's generously endowed with federal grants and private gifts. Most of this kind of money goes to research, but if they're going to keep the test tubes bubbling, it makes sense that they'll keep the lights on in the rest of the joint as well. This is a list of the institutions with the biggest research budgets in millions of dollars.

	In Millions
University of Pittsburgh School of Medicine, Pittsburgh, PA	$599
University of California School of Medicine San Francisco, CA	$250
Johns Hopkins University School of Medicine, Baltimore, MD	$239
Yale University School of Medicine, New Haven, CT	$203
University of Michigan Medical School, Ann Arbor, MI	$200
UCLA School of Medicine, Los Angeles, CA	$178
University of Alabama School of Medicine, Birmingham, AL	$175
University of Washington School of Medicine, Seattle, WA	$171
Baylor College of Medicine, Houston, TX	$163
Columbia University College of Physicians and Surgeons, New York, NY	$140
Mayo Medical School, Rochester, MN	$125
University of Chicago, Pritzker School of Medicine, Chicago, IL	$116
Duke University School of Medicine, Durham, NC	$107
Stanford University School of Medicine, Stanford, CA	$105
Vanderbilt University School of Medicine, Nashville, TN	$103
Georgetown University School of Medicine, Washington, DC	$100
University of California School of Medicine, San Diego, CA	$100
University of Iowa College of Medicine, Iowa City, IA	$100

MOST FINANCIAL AID

Don't get too excited. Most financial aid for would-be doctors comes in the form of loans, as in, "You will have to pay the money back." However, there are lots of grants and even some scholarships out there for those deserving individuals. Here are the schools with the highest percentages of students (two-thirds or more of the school's enrollment) receiving financial aid.

Eastern Virginia Medical School, Norfolk, VA	92%
Loyola University, Stritch School of Medicine, Chicago, IL	92%
University of Chicago, Pritzker School of Medicine, Chicago, IL	90%
University of Oklahoma College of Medicine, Oklahoma City, OK	89%
Boston University School of Medicine, Boston, MA	88%
Medical College of Pennsylvania, Philadelphia, PA	88%
Morehouse School of Medicine, Atlanta, GA	88%
Texas A&M University Health Science Center, College Station, TX	88%
University of Texas Medical School at San Antonio, TX	88%
University of Louisville School of Medicine, Louisville, KY	87%
University of Minnesota School of Medicine, Duluth, MN	87%
Wright State University School of Medicine, Dayton, OH	87%
Creighton University School of Medicine, Omaha, NE	84%
Louisiana State University School of Medicine, Shreveport	84%
Southern Illinois University School of Medicine, Springfield, IL	84%
Temple University School of Medicine, Philadelphia, PA	84%
University of Arizona College of Medicine, Tucson, AZ	84%
University of South Carolina School of Medicine, Columbia, SC	84%
University of South Dakota School of Medicine, Vermillion, SC	84%
Rush Medical College of Rush University, Chicago, IL	83%
University of California College of Medicine, Irvine, CA	83%

University of Nevada School of Medicine, Reno, NV	83%
University of Virginia School of Medicine, Charlottesville, VA	83%
Howard University College of Medicine, Washington, DC	82%
Stanford University School of Medicine, Stanford, CA	82%
University of Connecticut School of Medicine, Farmington, CT	82%
University of Medicine and Dentistry of New Jersey, Piscataway, NJ	82%
University of Miami School of Medicine, Miami, FL	82%
University of Washington School of Medicine, Seattle, WA	82%
Johns Hopkins University School of Medicine, Baltimore, MD	81%
Marshall University School of Medicine, Huntington, WV	81%
Mercer University School of Medicine, Macon, GA	81%
New York Medical College, Valhalla, NY	81%
Pennsylvania State University College of Medicine, Hershey, PA	81%
Wake Forest University, Bowman Gray School of Medicine, Winston-Salem, NC	81%
University of North Dakota School of Medicine, Grand Forks, ND	80%
Virginia Commonwealth University School of Medicine, Richmond, VA	80%
Case Western Reserve University School of Medicine, Cleveland, OH	79%
Finch University of Health Sciences Chicago Medical School, Chicago, IL	79%
Georgetown University School of Medicine, Washington, DC	79%
Mt. Sinai School of Medicine, New York, NY	79%
SUNY Health Science Center at Syracuse College of Medicine, Syracuse, NY	78%
University of California School of Medicine, San Diego	78%
University of Pennsylvania School of Medicine, Philadelphia, PA	78%
University of Kansas School of Medicine, Kansas City, KS	77%

University of Rochester School of Medicine and Dentistry, Rochester, NY	77%
Albany Medical College, Albany, NY	76%
University of Arkansas for Medical Sciences College of Medicine, Little Rock, AR	76%
University of Kentucky College of Medicine, Lexington, KY	76%
Dartmouth Medical School, Hanover, NH	74%
Northeastern Ohio Universities College of Medicine, Rootstown, OH	74%
University of Cincinnati College of Medicine, Cincinnati, OH	74%
University of Medicine and Dentistry of New Jersey, Newark, NJ	74%
University of Southern California School of Medicine, Los Angeles, CA	73%
East Carolina University School of Medicine, Greenville, NC	71%
Emory University School of Medicine, Atlanta, GA	71%
Thomas Jefferson University, Jefferson Medical College, Philadelphia, PA	71%
Tulane University School of Medicine, New Orleans, LA	71%
University of Alabama School of Medicine, Birmingham, AL	71%
University of Massachusetts Medical School, Worcester, MA	70%
University of Maryland School of Medicine, Baltimore, MD	69%
Yeshiva University, Albert Einstein College of Medicine, Bronx, NY	68%

STATES WITH THE GREATEST
NUMBER OF MEDICAL SCHOOLS

If, for some reason, you and your medical school do not have an imme-
diate chemistry, it would be good to live in a state where there are more
choices. We're talking about a place where a person could start again
after some minor mistake, an unavoidable altercation, or—God for-
bid!—a failure. For those of you who believe in second chances, here's a
list of the states that have the greatest number of medical schools.

New York	13
California	10
Pennsylvania	8
Texas	8
Illinois	7
Ohio	6
Missouri	6
Georgia	4
Florida	4
Massachusetts	4
North Carolina	4

ONE-HORSE TOWNS

States with the Fewest Medical Schools

There are five states without medical schools—that's a little frightening, especially if you live in one of those states and want to go to medical school. No in-state tuition for you. Quite a few others have only one school. If you need the in-state breaks and you've got only one choice and one chance, don't mess up. Pay attention.

Alaska	0
Delaware	0
Idaho	0
Montana	0
Wyoming	0
Arkansas	1
Colorado	1
Hawaii	1
Indiana	1
Kansas	1
Maine	1
Mississippi	1
Nevada	1
New Hampshire	1
New Mexico	1
North Dakota	1
Oklahoma	1
Oregon	1
Rhode Island	1
South Dakota	1
Utah	1
Vermont	1
Washington	1

PART 2

LIFESTYLE

· ·

"Nature's imagination, as Freeman Dyson likes to say, is richer than ours, and he speaks marvellingly of this richness in the physical and biological worlds, the endless diversity of physical forms and forms of life. For me, as a physician, nature's richness is to be studied in the phenomenon of health and disease, in the endless forms of individual adaptation by which the human organism, people, adapt and reconstruct themselves, faced with the challenges and vicissitudes of life.

"Defects, disorders, diseases, in this sense can play a paradoxical role by bringing out latent powers, developments, evolutions, forms of life that might never be seen, or even imaginable, in their absence.

"Thus while one may be horrified by the ravages of developmental disorders or diseases, one may see them as creative, too—for if they destroy particular paths, particular ways of doing things, they may force the nervous system into making other paths and ways, force on it an unexpected growth and evolution. This other side of development or disease is something I see, potentially, in almost every patient."

Oliver Sachs, M.D.
An Anthropologist on Mars
Knopf, 1995

f you're really going to do your best in medical school, you need the right atmosphere. Ambience is everything. How can you be expected to study if you're depressed because of the weather, or because you feel out of place? How will you be able to pay attention in class if you're worrying about getting a date for the weekend, and the pool of eligible date fodder is not exactly overwhelming? Your studies will absorb so much of your time that you can't afford to be bothered by avoidable environmental annoyances like speeding tickets, air pollution, and intemperate extremes of temperature. Of course, one person's distractions are opportunities for the next student. This chapter will help you fit your choice of medical school to your personal lifestyle, your likes and dislikes, and whether you prefer the boondocks or the big city—high life or low, gleaming or grimy.

MOST ELIGIBLE MEN

Would school just not be the same without an abundance of male company? In each medical school on the following list, men outnumber women by at least two to one. The percentage of male students follows the name of the school.

	Percentage of Males
Albany Medical College, Albany, NY	91%
Uniformed Services University School of Medicine, Bethesda, MD	79%
University of Health Science College of Osteopathic Medicine, Kansas City, MO	75%
Texas Tech Medical School, Lubbock, TX	73%
University of Utah School of Medicine, Salt Lake City, UT	71%
Kirksville College of Osteopathic Medicine, Kirksville, MO	71%
University of New England College of Osteopathic Medicine, Biddeford, ME	71%
Medical College of Georgia, Augusta, GA	69%

University of Mississippi School of Medicine, Jackson, MS	69%
Creighton University School of Medicine, Omaha, NE	67%
Louisiana State University School of Medicine, Shreveport, LA	67%
Midwestern University, Arizona College of Osteopathic Medicine, Glendale, AZ	68%
Marshall University School of Medicine, Huntington, WV	67%
Nova Southeastern University College of Osteopathic Medicine Fort Lauderdale, FL	67%
Wake Forest University, Bowman Gray School of Medicine, Winston-Salem, NC	66%
University of Alabama School of Medicine, Birmingham, AL	65%
University of Kentucky College of Medicine, Lexington, KY	65%
University of South Florida College of Medicine, Tampa, FL	65%
Vanderbilt Univesity School of Medicine, Nashville, TN	65%
Loma Linda University School of Medicine, Loma Linda, CA	64%

MOST ELIGIBLE WOMEN

In many medical schools, women are not even close to being equally represented. However, there is some hope. The playing field is much closer to even in some 40 institutions. That is to say, the ratio is nearly one to one. And in a very few schools, the percentage of women is a point or two higher than the male enrollment. The following is a list of medical schools where the percentages of men and women students is very close to fifty-fifty. The percentage listed represents the total female enrollment.

Percentage of Females

University of Hawaii, John A. Burns School of Medicine, Honolulu, HI	54%
Morehouse College School of Medicine, Atlanta, GA	53%
University of Arizona College of Medicine, Tuscon, AZ	52%
University of Missouri School of Medicine, Kansas City, MO	52%

University of Vermont School of Medicine, Burlington, VT	51%
East Carolina School of Medicine, Greenville, NC	50%
East Virginia Medical School, Norfolk, VA	50%
Medical College of Pennsylvania School of Medicine, Philadelphia, PA	50%
Rush Medical College of Rush University, Chicago, IL	50%
University of Connecticut School of Medicine, Farmington, CT	50%
University of Massachusetts Medical School, Worcester, MA	50%
Wright State University School of Medicine, Dayton, OH	50%
Case Western Reserve University School of Medicine, Cleveland, OH	49%
Cornell University Medical School, New York, NY	49%
Marshall University School of Medicine, Huntington, WV	49%
Albany Medical College, Albany, NY	48%
Brown University School of Medicine, Providence, RI	48%
Mt. Sinai School of Medicine, New York, NY	48%
University of California School of Medicine, San Francisco, CA	48%
University of Maryland School of Medicine, Baltimore, MD	48%

CULTURAL DIVERSITY

Schools with At Least a One-Fifth Minority Enrollment

Do you refuse to live in a monochromatic world? Is an ethnic mix of students of many cultures and colors important to your education? Then choose a school from the following list of schools, where minority students make up at least one-fifth of the enrollment.

Morehouse School of Medicine, Atlanta, GA	97%
Howard University College of Medicine, Washington, DC	90%
Meharry Medical College, Nashville, TN	86%

Nova Southeastern University College of Osteopathic Medicine, Fort Lauderdale, FL	66%
University of California College of Medicine, Irvine, CA	59%
Northwestern University Medical School, Chicago, IL	56%
Albany Medical College, Albany, NY	54%
University of Texas Medical School at Galveston, TX	47%
Midwestern University Chicago College of Osteopathic Medicine, Chicago, IL	40%
University of New Mexico School of Medicine, Albuquerque, NM	37%
Texas A&M University College of Medicine, College Station, TX	35%
Michigan State University College of Human Medicine, East Lansing, MI	34%
University of Medicine and Dentistry of New Jersey, School of Osteopathic Medicine, Stratford, NJ	33%
University of South Florida College of Medicine, Tampa	33%
Western University of Health Sciences, College of Osteopathic Medicine of the Pacific, Pomona, CA	33%
Pennsylvania State University College of Medicine, Hershey, PA	28%
UCLA School of Medicine, Los Angeles, CA	28%
Wright State University School of Medicine, Dayton, OH	28%
University of Illinois College of Medicine, Chicago, IL	27%
Ohio State University College of Medicine, Columbus, OH	26%
University of Texas Medical School, San Antonio, TX	26%
University of California School of Medicine, San Francisco, CA	24%
University of Cincinnati College of Medicine, Cincinnati, OH	24%
University of North Carolina School of Medicine, Chapel Hill, NC	24%
University of Texas Houston Medical School, Houston, TX	24%
Midwestern University Arizona College of Osteopathic Medicine, Glendale, AZ	22%
Texas Tech University Health Sciences Center School of Medicine, Lubbock, TX	22%

University of Medicine and Dentistry of New Jersey, Piscataway, NJ	21%
University of Oklahoma Medical School, Oklahoma City, OK	21%
Emory University School of Medicine, Atlanta, GA	20%
Harvard Medical School, Cambridge, MA	20%
New York Institute of Technology College of Osteopathic Medicine, Old Westbury, NY	20%
SUNY Health Science Center, Syracuse, NY	20%
Vanderbilt University School of Medicine, Nashville, TN	20%
Yale University School of Medicine, New Haven, CT	20%

LOWEST UNEMPLOYMENT

If you will be seeking full- or part-time work while attending medical school, or if you intend on settling near your school, an area with a strong job market is important. Here are the metropolitan areas with the lowest unemployment rates, and the schools nearby.

San Francisco, California

3.3% Plenty of work in this beautiful city, but finding an apartment might be something else.

University of California School of Medicine, San Francisco

Anaheim–Santa Ana, California

3.4% The hot spot in the Los Angeles basin.

University of California School of Medicine, Irvine

Washington, DC, and its suburbs

3.4% The United States government wants you.

George Washington University School of Medicine and Health Sciences

Georgetown University School of Medicine

Howard University College of Medicine

Uniformed Services University of the Health Sciences, Bethesda

Charlotte–Gastonia–Rock Hill, North Carolina and South Carolina

3.5.% Charlotte and environs remains a rapidly growing area.

Duke University School of Medicine, Durham

University of North Carolina at Chapel Hill School of Medicine

Seattle, Washington

3.5% The joke used to be, "Last guy out of Seattle, turn out the lights." But with the aerospace industry back on track, the lights stay on.

University of Washington School of Medicine, Seattle

Greensboro/Winston-Salem, North Carolina

3.7% Another growing part of a booming state.

Wake Forest University, Bowman Gray School of Medicine, Winston-Salem

Rochester, New York

3.7% They're saying "smile" over at Kodak.

University of Rochester School of Medicine and Dentistry

Milwaukee, Wisconsin

3.8% There must be something in the cheese. They are working in Wisconsin.

Medical College of Wisconsin, Milwaukee

University of Wisconsin Medical School, Madison

Nassau-Suffolk, New York

3.8% With the Atlantic Ocean in one direction and Long Island Sound to the north, it's surprising anyone works here at all.

SUNY Stony Brook School of Medicine Health Sciences Center

New York Institute of Technology College of Osteopathic Medicine, Old Westbury

Nashville, Tennessee

4% Did Dolly Parton's Dollywood contribute *that* many new jobs to the area?

Meharry Medical College School of Medicine, Nashville

Vanderbilt University School of Medicine, Nashville

Salt Lake City–Ogden, Utah

4.1% A sure sign a city is growing—they've got an NBA franchise in Salt Lake; but why did they call it the Jazz?

University of Utah School of Medicine, Salt Lake City

Cincinnati, Ohio

4.2% After years of stagnation, the Midwest is making headway again.

University of Cincinnati College of Medicine

Portland, Oregon

4.2% Portland is the new Seattle, ever since Seattle was overpublicized and overrun.

Oregon Health Sciences University School of Medicine, Portland

Minneapolis–St. Paul, Minnesota

4.3% Together, these two cities are doing twice as well as much of the surrounding countryside.

University of Minnesota Medical School, Minneapolis

Columbus, Ohio

4.4% In the past several years downtown Columbus has been rebuilt, and the state capital has become a magnet for regional corporate headquarters.

Ohio State University School of Medicine, Columbus

San Diego, California

4.5% The Silicon Valley of the south, San Diego continues to grow into the wireless communications capital of America.

University of California School of Medicine, San Diego

Denver, Colorado

4.6% If they can just keep that new airport open for a while, things might get even better here.

University of Colorado School of Medicine, Denver

Philadelphia, Pennsylvania

4.6% If you have your heart set on the Northeast, this is one of the few urban areas that hasn't been clobbered by unemployment.

Thomas Jefferson University, Jefferson Medical College, Philadelphia

Medical College of Pennsylvania and Hahnemann University School of Medicine, Philadelphia

University of Pennsylvania School of Medicine, Philadelphia

Temple University School of Medicine, Philadelphia

Philadelphia College of Osteopathic Medicine, Philadelphia

SCHOOLS IN THE STICKS

Does the frenzy of city life make you crazy? Do you like waking up to the scent of fresh air and a herd of cattle? Is walking that half mile out to your mail box, then hitting up Elsie for breakfast your idea of the perfect send off each morning? Then here is a list of medical schools on the rural route (or at least within hiking distance of the boondocks).

East Carolina University School of Medicine, Greenville, NC—Enjoy the Carolina countryside.

University of Missouri, Columbia School of Medicine, Columbia, MO— The first state university established west of the Mississippi, in 1839. There is still some frontier spirit here.

Kirksville College of Osteopathic Medicine, Kirksville, MO—At least Columbia is on the main drag between Kansas City and St. Louis. Kirksville is nearonly itself.

Mayo Medical School, Rochester, MN—Equidistant from the towns of Zumbrota, Owatonna, and LaCrosse.

Northeastern Ohio Universities College of Medicine, Rootstown, OH—Prime-time TV commercials in this area offer pesticides to corn farmers with rootworm problems.

Texas Tech University Health Sciences Center School of Medicine, Lubbock, TX—West Texas High Plains, home of the Blue Norther.

University of Florida College of Medicine, Gainesville, FL—A big small-town surrounded by cattle ranches, sink holes, clear springs, and year-ling country.

University of New England College of Osteopathic Medicine, Biddeford, ME—Between the rockbound coast and the endless cedar timberland.

West Virginia School of Osteopathic Medicine, Lewisberg, WV—This place is in the middle of the Allegheny Mountains in the Appalachian Range. We're talking big-time hills.

BIG CITY SCHOOLS

"How're you gonna keep 'em down on the ranch once they see Dallas?" If you like your air with a little texture and a few added minerals, or if you like living 20 or more stories above ground, then you might be a natural-born city slicker. This list is for those who want to be surrounded by a metropolitan area of a million inhabitants or more.

Atlanta

Emory University School of Medicine, Atlanta

Morehouse School of Medicine, Atlanta

Boston area

Boston University School of Medicine

Harvard Medical School

Tufts University School of Medicine

Chicago

University of Chicago, Pritzker School of Medicine

Finch University of Health Sciences, Chicago Medical School

University of Illinois College of Medicine

Loyola University of Chicago, Stritch School of Medicine

Northwestern University Medical School

Rush Medical College of Rush University

Dallas–Fort Worth

University of Texas Southwestern Medical Center at Dallas

University of North Texas Health Science Center College of Osteopathic Medicine, Fort Worth

Denver

University of Colorado School of Medcine

Houston

Baylor College of Medicine, Houston

University of Texas Houston Medical School

Los Angeles area

University of California College of Medicine, Irvine

UCLA School of Medicine, Los Angeles

University of Southern California School of Medicine, Los Angeles

Loma Linda University School of Medicine, Loma Linda

Western University of Health Sciences, College of Osteopathic Medicine of the Pacific, Pomona

Miami

University of Miami School of Medicine, Miami

Nova Southeastern University College of Osteopathic Medicine, Fort Lauderdale

New York

Yeshiva University, Albert Einstein College of Medicine, Bronx

Columbia University College of Physicians and Surgeons

Cornell University Medical College

Mount Sinai School of Medicine of the City University of New York

New York University School of Medicine

New York Medical College, Valhalla

SUNY Health Science Center at Brooklyn College of Medicine

Pittsburgh

University of Pittsburgh School of Medicine

Philadelphia

Thomas Jefferson University, Jefferson Medical College, Philadelphia

Medical College of Pennsylvania and Hahnemann University School of Medicine, Philadelphia

University of Pennsylvania School of Medicine, Philadelphia

Temple University School of Medicine, Philadelphia

Philadelphia College of Osteopathic Medicine, Philadelphia

San Francisco

University of California School of Medicine, San Francisco

Seattle

University of Washington School of Medicine

St. Louis

St. Louis University Health Sciences Center

Washington University School of Medicine, St. Louis

Washington, DC

George Washington University School of Medicine and Health Sciences

Georgetown University School of Medicine

Howard University College of Medicine

Crime Rates By Region

Though the rate of violent crime, burglary, larceny, and motor vehicle theft are all down dramatically in recent years (by 25 percent to 40 percent in most areas), some places are simply safer than others. Here is a list by region of the states with the highest crime rates in two categories, violent crimes and crimes against property. The figures represent the number of reported crimes per 100,000 residents. States with large, metropolitan areas generally have higher crime rates. You should also remember that although university campuses are not immune to crime, they are still safe havens from most violent behavior, even in the worst of cities. Also, remember that the statewide crime rate may be quite different from the rate in the community in which the school is located.

New England

	Violent Crimes	Crimes against Property
Massachusetts	687.2	3,654.4
Connecticut	405.9	4,097.3

(Connecticut's murder rate of 4.6 per 100,000 residents is the worst in New England, thanks to the influx of youth gangs in the state's cities.)

New Hampshire	114.5	2,540.9

(New Hampshire is the safest place in New England.)

Rhode Island	368	3,876.6

Middle Atlantic

New York	841.9	3,718.3

(For all its bad reputation because of New York City, property crimes are relatively low in New York State, and getting lower.)

New Jersey	599.8	4,103.9
Pennsylvania	427.3	2,937.6

Midwest

Illinois	996.1	4,459.6
Michigan	687.8	4,495
Indiana	524.7	4,106.8
Ohio	482.5	3,922.7
Wisconsin	281.1	3,604

(The least violent state in the area, by far.)

North Central

Missouri	663.8	4,456.8
Kansas	420.7	4,466.2
Nebraska	382	4,162.5

(This state is basically calm, but has been impacted by youth gangs.)

Minnesota	356.1	4,141.2
Iowa	354.4	3,747.5
South Dakota	207.5	2,853.1
North Dakota	86.7	2,779.6

(The least violent state in the nation.)

South

District of Columbia	2,661.4	9,512.1

(The nation's capital is far and a way the most violent and crime-ridden city in America. The murder rate is 65 per 100,000 residents. The next worst is in the teens.)

Florida	1,071	6,630.6
Louisiana	1,007.4	5,668.6

(Second highest murder rate: 17.2 per 100,000 residents)

Maryland	986.9	5,307.9
South Carolina	981.9	5,081

Tennessee	771.5	4,591.2
Georgia	657.1	5,346.5
North Carolina	646.4	4,993.1
Alabama	632.4	4,215.7
Arkansas	553.2	4,137.7
Mississippi	502.8	4,011.7

Virginia, West Virginia, and Kentucky all have violent crime rates below the 500 per 100,000 make. West Virginia's rate of violent crimes is down at 210.

West

Nevada	945.2	5,634.2
New Mexico	819.2	5,608.8
Arizona	713.5	7,500.1
Oklahoma	664.1	4,932
Texas	663.9	5,020
Colorado	440.2	4,956.1
Utah	328.8	5,762
Idaho	322	4,079.4
Wyoming	254.2	4,066
Montana	170.6	5,134.4

Pacific Coast

California	966	4,865.1
Alaska	770.9	4,982.9
Oregon	522.4	6,041.5
Washington	484.3	5,785.5
Hawaii	295.6	6,902.9

MOST ANNUAL PRECIPITATION

Does anyone like rain besides farmers and the folks at the Totes umbrella factory? You can't get a tan if it's raining all the time. If you can't get a tan, you won't look your best. If you don't look your best, you won't feel good. If you're not feeling good, you won't be thinking good, and that could really mess up your plans for a medical license. Most of the rain activity is concentrated in the Gulf Coast states, with a few exceptions scattered to the Northeast and Northwest. If you get depressed by light deprivation, and you hate wet feet, here are the schools to avoid.

Little Rock, Arkansas

It may have been more than ambition that drove President Clinton from Arkansas to Washington, DC. Little Rock experiences an average annual rainfall of 72 inches, the highest in the continental United States.

University of Arkansas for Medical Sciences College of Medicine, Little Rock

Florida

The Sunshine State sees plenty of H_2O, from Miami's whopping 55.91 inches a year to Jacksonville, where the ground stays pretty darn damp with 51.32 inches of rain annually. But take heart: Most of the rain, especially in the warmer months, occurs in the afternoon—every afternoon, and in buckets full. The daily deluge usually lasts no more than half an hour, then it's back to fun in the sun.

University of Florida College of Medicine, Gainesville

University of Miami School of Medicine, Miami

Nova Southeastern University College of Osteopathic Medicine, Fort Lauderdale

University of South Florida College of Medicine, Tampa

Mobile, Alabama

It rains in Mobile an average of more than an inch a week (63.96 inches annually), and it isn't much better upstate in Birmingham, where they average 54.6 inches a year. That's why there's more Spanish moss than people in Alabama.

University of Alabama School of Medicine, Birmingham

University of Southern Alabama College of Medicine, Mobile

Georgia

The Okefenokee Swamp near Waycross, GA, is not an aberration. It's representative of much of the state. It's not a big surprise that a low-lying coastal town like Savannah gets almost 50 inches of rain a year. But Atlanta is a little worse at 50.77 inches.

Emory University School of Medicine, Atlanta

Morehouse School of Medicine, Atlanta

Medical College of Georgia School of Medicine, Augusta

Mercer University School of Medicine, Macon

New Orleans, Louisiana

A cool town, a fun town, a really wet town. If you've been there, you've noticed that they bury people above ground because the water table is so high. New Orleans is almost underwater in any case, but it doesn't help that they get 61.88 inches of rain a year.

Louisiana State University School of Medicine in New Orleans

Tulane University School of Medicine, New Orleans

Galveston-Houston, Texas

They do things big in Texas. Galveston gets a saturating 42.28 inches of rain a year. But that's nothing compared to the weather they get in Houston: Tennis ball-sized hail and storms that could float Noah's Ark. It once rained out a baseball game at the Astrodome: The umpires couldn't get from their hotel to the stadium because of flooding.

Baylor College of Medicine, Houston

University of Texas Houston Medical School

University of Texas Medical School at Galveston

New York, New York

Many New Yorkers don't think of their city as having weather. But those who count the drops confirm that New York City drinks up a much-above-average 42.12 inches of annual rainfall. Albany and Buffalo upstate may brag because they get fewer inches a year, but most of theirs comes down as snow.

Yeshiva University, Albert Einstein College of Medicine, Bronx

Columbia University College of Physicians and Surgeons

Cornell University Medical College

Mount Sinai School of Medicine of the City University of New York

New York University School of Medicine

New York Medical College, Valhalla

SUNY Health Science Center at Brooklyn College of Medicine

SUNY Stony Brook School of Medicine Health Sciences Center

New York Institute of Technology College of Osteopathic Medicine, Old Westbury

University of Rochester School of Medicine and Dentistry

SUNY at Buffalo School of Medicine and Biomedical Sciences

SUNY Health Science Center at Syracuse College of Medicine

Albany Medical College, Albany

Seattle-Tacoma, Washington

For all its bad reputation as the rain and drizzle capitol of the nation, the Seattle-Tacoma area experiences a relatively moderate 37.19 inches of rain annually. The real problem is that, when it's not raining, it's cloudy. Sunshine is mostly a rumor in the Northwest.

University of Washington School of Medicine, Seattle

Phoenix, Arizona

No rain. At 7.66 inches of rain per year, they have the least precipitation of any major American city. If you see any spare rain around your neck of the woods, they'd appreciate your scooping it up in a pail and sending it to Phoenix today.

University of Arizona College of Medicine, Tucson

Midwestern University Arizona College of Osteopathic Medicine, Glendale

THE GOOD, THE NOT-SO-BAD, AND THE UGLY

Schools Listed by the Weather

Weatherwise, the following locations are the Good, the Not-So-Bad, and the Downright Ugly on the American landscape. The Good are places with the most temperate overall climates. The Not-So-Bad have a relatively moderate year with at least one horrendous season. The Ugly are places with flat-out crummy weather most of the year, excluding a few days here and there.

The Good

Honolulu, Hawaii

There is only one season in Hawaii—the gorgeous season. The January temperatures range between 66 and 80 degrees. July hovers between 74 and 88. The annual rainfall is only 22 inches, so this is paradise indeed.

University of Hawaii John A. Burns School of Medicine, Honolulu

San Diego, California

It is rarely too hot or too cold in Southern California. The average normal temperature in January ranges from 44 to 49 degrees, and in July the thermometer stays mostly between 66 and 76. With their scant 9.9 inches of annual rainfall, Southern California has one of the most temperate, sunny climates in the nation.

Los Angeles, California

Yes, there's the smog, but there's also a year-round mean temperature range of 49 to 84 degrees. Palm trees, oranges growing in your front yard—that's not too hard to take.

University of California College of Medicine, Irvine

UCLA School of Medicine, Los Angeles

University of Southern California School of Medicine, Los Angeles

Loma Linda University School of Medicine, Loma Linda

Western University of Health Sciences, College of Osteopathic Medicine of the Pacific, Pomona

University of California School of Medicine, San Diego

Albuquerque, New Mexico

Most of New Mexico shares the dry, clear air of neighboring Arizona and Nevada, but Albuquerque's altitude eliminates much of the searing summer heat. The normal winter average temperature is a brisk 22 to 47 degrees, but in that dry mountain air (there are fewer than nine inches of annual rainfall here) it is the mildest 22 degrees you will ever experience. The summer range is a moderate 67 to 93 degrees.

University of New Mexico School of Medicine

The Not-So-Bad

Maine

There's no denying the frigid Maine winter. The January temperature range in Portland is between a rather nasty 11 and 30 degrees. But for those who loathe hot weather, Maine is the place—they just don't have any. The temperatures in July range from 58 to 79 degrees. Anything over 80 is considered a heat wave.

University of New England College of Osteopathic Medicine, Biddeford, ME

Florida

Let's face it, the place is a steam bath in the summer. But ah, those South Florida winters that the retirees are so crazy for. For instance, the average winter temperatures in Miami range from 59 to 75 degrees. The Gulf Stream allows only a few freak freezes south of Orlando every five years or so. But don't trust those sunny brochures from schools in the northern half of the state—it gets almost as cold as Atlanta in Jacksonville, Gainesville, and Tallahassee.

University of Miami School of Medicine, Miami

Nova Southeastern University College of Osteopathic Medicine, Fort Lauderdale

University of South Florida College of Medicine, Tampa

Tucson, Arizona

Dry air notwithstanding, you'd have to be a lizard to wake up looking forward to a 106-degree summer day. But January is a totally different story. The winter temperatures have been recorded in the teens in New Mexico, but you could live another hundred years and not see it happen. The normal winter temperature range is between 41 and 66 degrees.

University of Arizona College of Medicine, Tucson

Midwestern University Arizona College of Osteopathic Medicine, Glendale

Portland, Oregon

It's wet and dismal during the winter rainy season, with the mean temperature squatting between 34 and 45 degrees. But summers are dry and moderate, more like spring extended to September or October.

Oregon Health Sciences University School of Medicine, Portland

The Ugly

The High Plains

Extending through parts of 13 states from the Dakotas down through the Texas panhandle south to Mexico, the High Plains were once called the Great American Desert. It starts where the rain ends in the East at about the 98th meridian. Forest gives way to grasslands and then to sage brush. The harsh weather anvil stretches all the way to the foothills of the Rocky Mountains and Denver. With long, hot summers and longer, freezing winters, this area makes up one-fifth of the land mass of the continental United States. St. Louis, Missouri, is the gateway city to the Plains, and that anyone lives there is proof that Missourians are stubborn. The January temperature range is a wintry 21 to 38 degrees, and it's a rare summer that the mercury doesn't hit 100. Parts of Texas, Oklahoma, Kansas, Nebraska, North and South Dakota (they don't call it the badlands for nothing) are included in the High Plains and the generally intemperate weather.

St. Louis University Health Sciences Center

Washington University School of Medicine, St. Louis

University of Missouri, Columbia School of Medicine

University of Missouri, Kansas City School of Medicine

University of Health Sciences College of Osteopathic Medicine, Kansas City

Kirksville College of Osteopathic Medicine, Kirksville

Texas Tech University Health Science Center School of Medicine, Lubbock

University of Oklahoma College of Medicine, Oklahoma City

University of North Dakota School of Medicine, Grand Forks

University of South Dakota School of Medicine, Vermillion

Creighton University School of Medicine, Omaha

University of Nebraska School of Medicine, Omaha

University of Kansas School of Medicine, Kansas City

ALL THE HELP YOU CAN GET

Schools with Religious Affiliations

Just as there are no atheists in foxholes, almost all medical students say a little prayer before every examination. If you think having a direct conduit to the religion of your choice might make a difference in your grade point average or at least in your sense of well being, here is a list of medical schools with religious affiliations. None of them limits enrollment to their own persuasion.

Baylor University College of Medicine, Houston, TX (Baptist)

Creighton University School of Medicine, Omaha, NE (Catholic)

Duke University School of Medicine, Durham, NC (Methodist)

Emory University School of Medicine, Atlanta, GA (Methodist)

Georgetown University School of Medicine, Washington, DC (Catholic)

Loma Linda University School of Medicine, Loma Linda, CA (Seventh Day Adventist)

Loyola University of Chicago, Stritch School of Medicine, Chicago, IL (Catholic)

St. Louis University School of Medicine, St. Louis, MO (Catholic)

Yeshiva University, Albert Einstein School of Medicine, New York, NY (Jewish)

PART 3

ENTERTAINMENT VALUE

"The most dramatic experience I have ever heard described of the apparent conscious control of internal or vegetative functions was seen repeatedly in the late 1950s by young doctors training at a famous university hospital. Told to me by a colleague . . ., the story involves a man in his forties who made a habit of turning up in the emergency room with one or another complaint. He would sit in a conspicuous part of the waiting area and promptly fall unconscious onto the floor. When the doctors rushed to his side, they would invariably find him to be without a pulse and not breathing—in cardiac arrest and turning bluer by the second. Because he always responded in less than a minute to resuscitation efforts, it never became necessary to jolt his heart with electricity or to go very far with that era's predecessor to CPR; although he had multiple surgical scars on various parts of his trunk, they were not of the sort through which the chest might have been opened for cardiac massage.

"The young doctors never noticed that none of the participating nurses seemed particularly alarmed by the life threatening drama taking place before their eyes . . . They were in on a scam they had seen many times before.

"The patient seemed to know when a new group of vice doctors was scheduled to begin the standard four to six week training rotation through the emergency room, and he would time his stunt for one of the first days after they arrived."

Sherwin B. Nuland, M.D.
The Wisdom of the Body
Knopf, 1997

Attending medical school is a very serious pursuit. Academics is in the forefront of everyone's mind who is struggling toward an M.D. But let's face it, you can't think about metatarsals, amino acids, calculus, and inorganic chemistry all the time. It would drive you nuts. All that assembly and disassembly of pieces over and over would send even the sanest person around the bend sooner or later.

If you're going to perform at your peak in medical school, and if you're going to justify your investment in tuition and all your early years of education, then you've got to make sure you get a minimum weekly allowance of undiluted fun and diversion. Obviously, it is imperative that you choose a school that allows you to partake in essential personal fun, either by providing the fun or being located in the proximity of fun and diversion. This chapter highlights some major sources of real big fun and lists the schools within easy striking distance. Hopefully you'll find your favorite kinds of fun here, use the information to make the right school choice, and totally avoid ending up gibbering to yourself and drooling all over your sweat-stained hospital gown. Take a few minutes today to protect yourself and your future by making sure you can collect your fair share of fun in an organized and regular fashion.

NEAR THE BEACH

When the going gets tough, do you just want to go to the beach? You're not alone. Sand and surf is a restorative for the soul, and the following areas provide some of the most perfect sand you'll ever get in your bathing suit. If you think the two most perfect words in the English language are "Surf's up!" pick your school from the following list.

New York

Some of the most beautiful beaches in the country are found on the south shore of Long Island, **New York,** beginning at Long Beach and running East through Jones Beach, Robert Moses State Park, Fire Island, The Hamptons, Amagansett, and all the way to the lighthouse on Montauk Point. The swimming is great, and the people watching is even better—male and female bathing beauties of every nationality in the world throng to these beaches from the New York City metropolitan area. Under rarely experienced optimum conditions, the drive from Manhattan to Jones Beach State Park is a mere 45 minutes. Better to count on an hour-and-a-half commute each way.

On Long Island within 30 to 45 minutes of the beach:

SUNY at Stony Brook Health Science Center, Stony Brook, NY

New York Institute of Technology College of Osteopathic Medicine, Old Westbury, NY

In the city within the 90-minute range of surf and sand:

Columbia University College of Physicians and Surgeons

Cornell University Medical School

Mount Sinai School of Medicine

New York University School of Medicine

SUNY at Brooklyn Health Science Center

Yeshiva University, Albert Einstein School of Medicine, Bronx, NY

Boston

If you can handle the frigid temperatures of the North Atlantic surf, consider schools in the **Boston** area. Nearby the city are the beaches of Duxbury and Whitehorse. Within a few hours' drive are the graceful dunes and roaring waves of Cape Cod. Beyond the Cape, by ferry or small plane, are the island playgrounds of the rich and celebrated, Martha's Vineyard and Nantucket Island.

Boston University School of Medicine

Harvard Medical School, Cambridge

Tufts University School of Medicine

University of Massachusetts Medical School

New Jersey

The **New Jersey** Shore stretches for over 100 miles from Atlantic Highlands to Cape May. The farther south you go, the wider the sandy beaches become and the better the swimming and surfing. The choice locations are in the vicinity of Atlantic City—perhaps the birthplace of the American boardwalk. But if you like your salt air tinged with the smell of hot dogs and the hurdy-gurdy sound of the Ferris wheel wafting on the ocean breeze, visit the slightly seedy Asbury Park. You can make it to the beach in an hour, even from Philadelphia, via the Atlantic City Expressway.

University of Medicine and Dentistry of New Jersey, Newark

University of Medicine and Dentistry of New Jersey, Piscataway

Maryland and Virginia

You've got to really want to get to the beach to reach Ocean City, **Maryland,** and the Eastern Shore of **Virginia**, but these are some great summer retreats. The islands of Assateague and Chincoteague—once you get away from the motels—are filled with wildlife, seabirds, and miles of unoccupied sand. If you get tired of lying in the sun, you can take a day trip by ferry into the Chesapeake Bay to Smith Island or the more remote Tangier Island for the best blue crab in the world. These are the beaches that serve the **Baltimore-Washington, DC**, chunk of the East Coast megalopolis.

George Washington University School of Medicine and Health Sciences

Georgetown University School of Medicine

Howard University College of Medicine

Uniformed Services University of the Health Sciences, Bethesda

Johns Hopkins School of Medicine, Baltimore

University of Maryland School of Medicine, Baltimore

Virginia Beach and North Carolina

Virginia Beach to the north and Myrtle Beach to the south flank the Outer Banks of **North Carolina** are like two gaudy rhinestone clasps on the ends of a string of pearl-like beaches. The places in between are a national treasure: The wide dunes and pristine sands of these barrier islands are as unsullied as the neon-tinged, high-rise-pocked cities of Virginia Beach and Myrtle Beach are overbuilt and overrun. On the Outer Banks, you can roam the beaches where Blackbeard may have hidden his treasure. Just the names of places evoke the mystery of the sea and the adventure of sailing in the long-distant past: Cape Lookout, Cape Fear. One of the quaint island towns to spend time in is Okracoke, with its squat white lighthouse. Plus it's a ferry port, in case you do get the urge to play Goofy Golf on a three-story miniature golf course with a bright turquoise waterfall tumbling over an imitation of the Pyramid of Giza.

Eastern Virginia Medical School of the Medical College of Hampton Roads, Norfolk

East Carolina University School of Medicine, Greenville

Schools within a few hours of these beaches:

Virginia Commonwealth University Medical College, Richmond

University of Virginia School of Medicine, Charlottesville

Bowman Gray School of Medicine of Wake Forest University, Winston-Salem

Duke University School of Medicine, Durham

University of North Carolina at Chapel Hill School of Medicine

Medical University of South Carolina College of Medicine, Charleston

University of South Carolina School of Medicine, Columbia

Florida

Florida is one big sand bar sticking out into the water between the Atlantic ocean and the Gulf of Mexico. Here you can experience every kind of beach atmosphere in one state—the tacky urbanism at South Beach in Miami; rugged and isolated surf along the northeast coast near St. Augustine, Jacksonville, and Fernandina; the retirees' dream of sugar-white sand and warm-as-weak-tea water in Clearwater, St. Pete, and in the panhandle at Pensacola. In Key West, you can stand where Hemingway may have stood looking at the confluence of the Ocean and the Gulf. Perhaps the only bad thing about going to school in Florida is that there's no better place to go for Spring Break.

University of Florida College of Medicine, Gainesville

University of Miami School of Medicine, Miami

Nova Southeastern University College of Osteopathic Medicine, Fort Lauderdale, FL

University of South Florida College of Medicine, Tampa

California

America's other ocean lover's paradise is **California**. Many of the state's schools are within a few hours' drive of the Pacific. While there is great, scenic splendor in the northern reaches—remarkable places like Big Sur and the rest of the Monterey Peninsula, Point Reyes, and Bodega Bay— the best beaches for frolicking in the waves without the protection of a wet suit are in Southern California, especially the San Diego area. The surf just gets better from there all the way down the Baja into Mexico. But if you prefer your beaches with an urban twist, there are Malibu, Venice Beach, and Santa Monica in L.A. and the place some people are calling neo-L.A., Santa Barbara.

University of California School of Medicine, Davis

University of California College of Medicine, Irvine

UCLA School of Medicine, Los Angeles

University of Southern California School of Medicine, Los Angeles

University of California School of Medicine, San Diego

University of California School of Medicine, San Francisco

Loma Linda University School of Medicine, Loma Linda

Stanford University School of Medicine, Stanford

Western University of Health Sciences College of Osteopathic Medicine of the Pacific, Pomona

Hawaii

The last word in beaches is **Hawaii**. What more can be said, except to apply early: the University of Hawaii, John A. Burns School of Medicine is taking just 56 students—and only three of them will be from out of state.

NEAR GREAT SKIING

The first skis, found preserved in bogs in Scandinavia and estimated to be 4,000 to 5,000 years old, were made from the large bones of extinct mammals. There's still something about mamboing down the fall line in deep powder that brings out the animal in human beings. Skiing is the closest thing to flying that a human being is capable of doing without leaving the ground. If you believe that a day spent on the slopes beats a day in classes any day of the week, then here are the schools for you.

Colorado

There's no competition. Colorado has more and better skiing than any other state in the Union. Just the names of the ski areas read like a snow mantra: Aspen, Snowmass, Vail, Keystone, Breckenridge, Copper Mountain, Steamboat Springs, Telluride, Monarch, Crested Butte, Glenwood, Durango, Purgatory. And there are 20 more lesser known ski slopes sprinkled through the Rocky Mountains, which dominate the landscape. The snow is deep and powdery from at least mid-November until the late spring. If you like to strap sticks to your feet and slide down hills, come to Colorado.

University of Colorado School of Medicine, Denver

Park City, Utah

Park City will be the site of the Winter Olympics in 2002. Get to school in the area immediately before the crowds of international rubberneckers beat the entire state into slush. Park City was probably the best undiscovered ski area in the nation until recent publicity about the worldwide competition descended on the village. The town is quaint, homey, graced with a gorgeous, 19th-century lodge, and the best—perhaps the only—sushi restaurant in Utah.

University of Utah School of Medicine, Salt Lake City

Sun Valley, Idaho

The very first ski resort was developed in Sun Valley in 1936 by the Union Pacific Railroad. The owners installed the first successful chair lift on Dollar Mountain, and the rest is skiing history. Sun Valley is still a magical place to leave a few sitzmarks in the snow. The town itself, with a population of only 938, sits at an elevation of 6,000 feet, overlooking a pristine Alpine landscape locked in geological time—not much has changed in the 60-odd years since Sun Valley opened to the public. However, you're going to have to fly to Sun Valley, since there are no medical schools in Idaho . . . or Wyoming, or Montana. The closest schools are in Nevada, Utah, Washington, and Oregon—each with one school.

University of Nevada School of Medicine, Reno

University of Utah School of Medicine, Salt Lake City

University of Washington School of Medicine, Seattle

Oregon Health Sciences University, Portland

Vermont

The Green Mountains form the granite backbone of this state. With only 9,600 square miles in Vermont, there are still 24 alpine ski areas, including Killington, Stowe, Okemo, Stratton Mountain, West Dover, Warren, and Burlington. Perhaps no other state has been so untouched by the developers' bulldozer blades and industrial pollution as Vermont. Despite temperatures that can dip well below zero, and the tendency of the local deep freeze to foster icy conditions on the slopes, Vermont consistently provides the best skiing in the East.

University of Vermont College of Medicine, Burlington

NEAR GREAT ZOOS AND AQUARIUMS

Reconnecting with our neighbors on this planet is good for the spirit. Face to face with the animals displaced with our so-called civilization, you may find your world view forced into a different perspective. Not only is contact with the animal kingdom soothing for the soul, there is much to learn from the beasts. When you're feeling the stress of credit overload, there's no better way to relieve the tension than to bop down to the zoo and talk it over with Dumbo. Or push your luck by making extended, syncopated eye contact with that marvelous killing machine, the Great White, as he circles around and around at the aquarium. Here are the best places to talk to the animals in America, followed by the number of annual visitors at each and the nearby graduate schools.

	Annual Visitors
Sea World of Florida, Orlando	4,000,000

University of Florida College of Medicine, Gainesville

University of Miami School of Medicine, Miami

Nova Southeastern University College of Osteopathic Medicine, North Miami Beach

University of South Florida College of Medicine, Tampa

Lincoln Park Zoological Gardens, Chicago, IL	4,000,000
John G. Shedd Aquarium, Chicago, IL	2,186,075
Chicago Zoological Park, Brookfield, IL	2,000,000

University of Chicago, Pritzker School of Medicine

Finch University of Health Sciences, Chicago
Medical School

University of Illinois College of Medicine

Loyola University, Chicago Stritch School of Medicine

Northwestern University Medical School

Rush Medical College of Rush University

San Diego Zoo, San Diego, CA	3,400,000
Sea World of California, San Diego, CA	3,000,000
San Diego Wild Animal Park, San Diego, CA	300,000

University of California School of Medicine, San Diego

National Zoological Park, Washington, DC	3,000,000

George Washington University School of Medicine
and Health Sciences

Georgetown University School of Medicine

Howard University College of Medicine

Uniformed Services University of the Health
Sciences, Bethesda

Busch Gardens, Tampa, FL	3,000,000

University of South Florida College of
Medicine, Tampa

St. Louis Zoological Park, St. Louis, MO	2,800,000

St. Louis University Health Sciences Center

Washington University School of Medicine, St. Louis

New York Zoological Park, Bronx, NY	2,000,000

Yeshiva University, Albert Einstein College of
Medicine, Bronx

Los Angeles Zoo, Los Angeles, CA	1,800,000

University of California College of Medicine, Irvine

UCLA School of Medicine, Los Angeles

University of Southern California School of Medicine,
Los Angeles

Loma Linda University School of Medicine,
Loma Linda

Western University of Health Sciences College
of Osteopathic Medicine of the Pacific, Pomona

Monterey Bay Aquarium, Monterey, CA   1,700,000

Stanford University School of Medicine, Stanford

National Aquarium, Baltimore, MD   1,500,000

Johns Hopkins School of Medicine

University of Maryland School of Medicine

Uniformed Services University of the Health
Sciences, Bethesda

Marine World Africa USA, Vallejo, CA   1,454,000

San Francisco Zoological Gardens, San Francisco, CA   1,000,000

University of California School of Medicine,
San Francisco

Milwaukee Zoological Gardens, WI   1,400,000

Medical College Wisconsin, Milwaukee

University of Wisconsin Medical School, Madison

Houston Zoological Gardens, Houston, TX   1,300,000

Baylor College of Medicine, Houston

University of Texas Houston Medical School

University of Texas Medical School at Galveston

Philadelphia Zoological Gardens, Philadelphia, PA   1,300,000

Thomas Jefferson University, Jefferson Medical College,
Philadelphia

Medical College of Pennsylvania and Hahnemann
University School of Medicine, Philadelphia

University of Pennsylvania School of
Medicine, Philadelphia

Temple University School of Medicine, Philadelphia

Philadelphia College of Osteopathic
Medicine, Philadelphia

New England Aquarium, Boston, MA   1,300,000

Boston University School of Medicine

Harvard Medical School, Cambridge

Tufts University School of Medicine

Denver Zoological Gardens, Denver, CO   1,300,000

University of Colorado School of Medicine, Denver

Cincinnati Zoo, Cincinnati, OH   1,287,000

University of Cincinnati College of Medicine

Minnesota Zoological Gardens, Apple Valley, MN   1,164,000

Mayo Medical School, Rochester

University of Minnesota, Duluth School of Medicine

University of Minnesota Medical School, Minneapolis

Sea World of Texas, San Antonio, TX   1,000,000

University of Texas Medical School at San Antonio

Metro Washington Park Zoo, Portland, OR   1,000,000

Oregon Health Sciences University School of
Medicine, Portland

Sea World of Ohio, Aurora, OH   1,000,000

Case Western Reserve University School of
Medicine, Cleveland

University of Cincinnati College of Medicine

Medical College of Ohio, Toledo

Northeastern Ohio Universities College of
Medicine, Rootsville

Ohio State University College of Medicine, Columbus

Wright State University School of Medicine, Dayton

NEAR GREAT ROLLER COASTERS

There is no better practice for the ups and downs of life than to ride the nation's great roller coasters. The first version of this amusement park ride that would be recognizable as a roller coaster was the Russian Mountains, built in Paris in 1804 as a carriage running on an inclined track. It was an adaptation of timbered slides covered with ice—some as high as 70 feet—that had been built in Russia for public entertainment since at least 1650. A giant, wood-framed roller coaster became the legendary centerpiece of New York City's Coney Island, and similar rides soon spread to oceanfront boardwalks on both coasts. The last few years have seen a renaissance in the art of building roller coasters, with new materials and technology sending the industry into overdrive. Oddly enough, the American city with the most roller coasters per capita today is Las Vegas, as the gambling casinos branch out to grab the family vacation dollar. What a combination—craps, slots, poker, and roller coasters. If that's your pleasure, consider the University of Nevada in Lost Wages. And here are some other great local rides and the universities attached to them.

1. MONTU at Busch Gardens, Tampa, Florida. The world's tallest and longest inverted coaster is named after a hawk-headed, human-bodied Egyptian warrior god. The first vertical loop stands 104 feet tall and is followed by another six inversions. Track length is approximately 3,983 feet with a top speed of 60 miles per hour. Maximum drop is 128 feet. Ride duration, approximately three minutes.

University of South Florida College of Medicine, Tampa

2. LOCH NESS MONSTER at Busch Gardens, Williamsburg, Virginia. This steel, interlocking-loop coaster with two inversions is 130 feet tall. After an initial drop of 114.2 feet, the cars are going 60 mph for a running time of 2 minutes, 10 seconds.

Eastern Virginia Medical School of the Medical College of Hampton Roads, Norfolk

University of Virginia School of Medicine, Charlottesville

3. OUTER LIMITS: FLIGHT OF FEAR located at both Kings Island in Cincinnati, Ohio and Kings Dominion, Richmond, Virginia. The ride is experienced entirely in the dark. There is no chain lift. Escape velocity is attained via an electromagnetic wave that carries you from zero to 55 mph in 3.9 seconds. The track length is 2,705 feet.

University of Cincinnati College of Medicine, OH

Virginia Commonwealth University Medical College, Richmond

4. WILD THING at Valleyfair, Shakoppe, Minnesota. Wild Thing is billed as one of the longest, tallest, and wildest rides in the world. It's 200 feet tall and more than a mile long. Cars will reach speeds up to 74 miles per hour. Hold onto your hat!

Mayo Medical School, Rochester

University of Minnesota, Duluth School of Medicine

University of Minnesota Medical School, Minneapolis

5. SUPERMAN THE ESCAPE at Six Flags Magic Mountain, Valencia, California. This is a state-of-the-art, gigantic L-shaped coaster. Vehicles blast out of the station, accelerating from 0 to 102 mph in seven seconds, and then shoot straight up the 41-story tower. The dual-track coaster spans more than 900 feet across the theme park, as much as 415 feet above the ground. The total track length is 1,235 feet.

University of California School of Medicine, San Francisco

Stanford University School of Medicine, Stanford

NEAR GREAT MALLS

Back in the 1920s Calvin Coolidge said, "The business of America is business." Well, the business of America is now shopping, and business is conducted at the mall. Malls began replacing Main Street in the early 1960s. Today, there are literally thousands of these concentrated shopping centers across the land. Here are the megamalls for those of you who suffer withdrawal symptoms if you don't shop every day.

Atlanta, Georgia.

The expression "shop till you drop" takes on an epic quality in Atlanta, which boasts no fewer than 11 malls in the metro area. You can warm up at the Cumberland Mall with its 145 stores on 72 acres; then try the Lenox Square on for size—212 stores on 63 acres of land. Better mark where you park here—the lot holds 7,000 cars.

Emory University School of Medicine, Atlanta

Morehouse School of Medicine, Atlanta

Baltimore, Maryland

You can start at Eastpoint Mall (152 stores), then sink your teeth into Metro Plaza, where there are another 125 businesses.

Johns Hopkins School of Medicine

University of Maryland School of Medicine

Bloomington, Minnesota

Here, just outside of the Twin Cities, resides the mother of all malls: The Mall of America. We're talking 500 stores! There are 66 restaurants, 29 woman's wear emporiums, 35 of what they call "unisex family clothing stores," and 13 different places that want to sell you jewelry. The only thing the place lacks on its 72 acres is a hotel—which you might need if you plan to traverse the entire place. But they're talking about expanding, so maybe that's next.

University of Minnesota Medical School, Minneapolis

Chicago, Illinois

Ford City's 142 stores are scattered over a whopping 100 acres.

University of Chicago, Pritzker School of Medicine

Finch University of Health Sciences, Chicago Medical School

University of Illinois College of Medicine

Loyola University, Chicago Stritch School of Medicine

Northwestern University Medical School

Rush Medical College of Rush University

Dallas, Texas

They do things big in Texas. Galleria Dallas packs 200 stores onto 43 acres. And if you can't find it here, there are seven other malls in town.

University of Texas Southwestern Medical Center at Dallas

University of North Texas Health Science Center College of Osteopathic Medicine, Fort Worth

Denver, Colorado

Working the Cherry Creek and Crossroads Malls could give you a Rocky Mountain shopping high, not to mention coronary arrest. Between them there are 320 stores on 102 acres.

University of Colorado School of Medicine, Denver

Jacksonville, Florida

Some people have entered the Avenues Mall and never been heard from again: 150 stores on 200 acres. Maybe they're looking for their cars in the 6,000 car lot. Or maybe they're over in Regency Square, where there are 170 more stores on 123 acres.

University of Florida College of Medicine, Gainesville

Miami, Florida

Mall-wise, Miami is the eye of the Florida shopping hurricane. There are 17 malls in the metro area. Three of them—Cutler Ridge, Dadeland, and Miami Intermall—have nearly 500 stores between them.

University of Miami School of Medicine, Miami

Nova Southeastern University College of Osteopathic Medicine, North Miami Beach

Houston, Texas

You think Dallas is something? Try The Galleria Houston version—310 stores. Oh, and there are another 15 malls in this city, too.

Baylor College of Medicine, Houston

University of Texas Houston Medical School

University of Texas Medical School at Galveston

Los Angeles, California

Do they mall-shop in L.A.? Try the Beverly Center, which crams 200 stores into eight acres. No luck? How about Century City, where there's another 140 stores. There are four other malls as well, but we're not going to tell you about them—you don't have enough money.

UCLA School of Medicine, Los Angeles

University of Southern California School of Medicine, Los Angeles

Omaha, Nebraska

The locals take their prairie dollars over to Westroads Mall, where there are 200 stores on 60 acres.

University of Nebraska College of Medicine, Omaha

Creighton University School of Medicine, Omaha

Orange County, California

Why drive to L.A. when there are 200 stores at Fashion Island?

University of California School of Medicine, Irvine

San Diego, California

The city is fortified by nine malls. Foremost among them is Fashion Valley Center, laden with the temptations of 148 stores.

University of California School of Medicine, San Diego

San Francisco, California

If you can't find anything in your size in Embarcardo Centers' 150 stores, you can always drive five miles south to Stonetown Galleria, where there are 160 more wallet-emptying enterprises.

University of California School of Medicine, San Francisco

NEAR NATURAL WONDERS

The beauty of nature is an inspiration. The serenity and peace of the wilderness can sustain your flagging spirits and repair the frayed edges of your intellect and emotions. Everybody needs a tree to hug. Here are graduate schools for nature lovers.

Boston, Massachusetts area

While there are no marquee natural attractions in Boston, there are three federally protected areas nearby: Great Meadows National Wildlife Reserve, Massosoit National Wildlife Reserve, and Parker River National Wildlife Reserve. Plus, there are no fewer than 31 separate state recreation areas in striking distance of the city.

Boston University School of Medicine

Harvard Medical School, Cambridge

Tufts University School of Medicine

University of Massachusetts School of Medicine, Worcester

Denver, Colorado

Denver definitely has its urban problems, including pollution, over-crowding, and traffic jams that are beginning to rival those in Los

Angeles. But, nestled in the shadow of the Rocky Mountains, Denver is just a hop, skip, and a jump from the Continental Divide, where the scenery is spectacular. The 27,000 acre Rocky Mountain National Park is within an easy commute. Besides, almost every square inch of the state west of Denver is a national forest.

University of Colorado School of Medicine, Denver

Central California

There is no place in the nation adorned by more natural splendor. There are six federally protected areas, including Yosemite National Park, Sequoia National Forest, Sierra National Forest, Inyo Canyon National Park, Devils Postpile National Forest, and Kings Canyon National Park. The medical school closest to all this wonder is outside Sacramento. So on the weekends, you can drive past the lettuce fields and into the hills.

University of California School of Medicine, Davis

Honolulu, Hawaii

This island is surrounded by 135 miles of Pacific Ocean coastline and some of the finest weather on the planet. There's also the 1,900 acre Hawaiian Islands National Wildlife Reserve.

University of Hawaii John A. Burns School of Medicine

Reno, Nevada

There are other reasons to live in Nevada besides Wayne Newton, dry air, and cheap housing. There are no fewer than eight federally protected natural areas in the vicinity, including such heavyweights as the Grand Canyon, Death Valley National Monument, and the 1,385,000 acre Lake Mead National Recreation Area.

University of Nevada School of Medicine, Reno

Long Island, New York

The attraction here is salt water. The Fire Island National Seashore is truly something special—that is, when hurricanes aren't washing away the beach and a few hundred houses at a time. This narrow island is a haven for dune and sea life, and is only a few short miles away from the East Coast megalopolis. There are also three National Wildlife Reserves on Long Island and Jones Beach State Park—a world class ocean beach.

SUNY Health Science Center at Brooklyn College of Medicine

SUNY Stony Brook School of Medicine Health Sciences Center

New York Institute of Technology College of Osteopathic Medicine, Old Westbury

Miami, Florida

There are plenty of gangsters and little old ladies with blue hair, but there are also 84 miles of Atlantic Ocean coastline, plus the eerie, enormous Everglades National Park. And don't forget the nearby fishing, snorkeling, and scuba diving offered by the Florida Keys.

University of Miami School of Medicine, Miami

Nova Southeastern University College of Osteopathic Medicine, North Miami Beach

Portland, Oregon

Besides the gigantic Mt. Hood National Forest (614,000 acres), the Siuslaw National Forest, and 11 State Recreation Areas, a relatively short ride lands you in the venerable Redwood National Forest.

Oregon Health Services University School of Medicine, Portland

Rapid City, South Dakota

Besides the man-made monument to dead presidents, Mt. Rushmore, there's the starkly beautiful Badlands National Park and the Black Hills National Forest (395,000 acres).

University of South Dakota School of Medicine, Vermillion

Tucson, Arizona

The Grand Canyon is in the same state, and there are five other federally protected areas in proximity of Tucson, most notably Cabeza Prieta

National Wildlife Reserve (416,000 acres) and the Organ Pipe Cactus National Monument (329,000 acres).

University of Arizona College of Medicine, Tucson

Seattle–Bellevue, Washington

It rains here 160 days a year on average. However, there's still great natural beauty to be seen through the mist: Mount Baker, Snoqualmie National Forests, and, 70 miles away, Olympic National Park.

University of Washington School of Medicine, Seattle

NEAR GREAT MICROBREWERIES

As all good med students know, if there is one essential nutrient all students need, it's beer. But not just any beer, and certainly not in a can—unless of course, nothing else is available or you've run out of cash and Bud Light is on sale for $4.59 a six-pack. No, the nation is being festooned with small beer breweries, marketing an incredible array of individualistic brews. If hops are your passion, and you care more about your beer's taste and character than its personality-altering effects when imbibed in mass quantities, the accessibility of microbreweries and their accompanying pubs should be factored into your search for the right school.

Boston–Cambridge

1. Back Bay Brewing Co. (established 1995)
   755 Boylston Street, Boston
   (617) 424-8300
   This brewpub offers brews with a historical theme.
   Types of brew: 5 regulars, 1 seasonal
   Food style: funky World Cuisine

2. Boston Beer Works (established 1992)
   61 Brookline Avenue, Boston (across from Fenway Park)
   (617) 536-2337

This is the largest brewpub (brewing volume) east of the Rockies.
Types of brew: 12 regulars, 2 seasonal
Food style: eclectic American

3. Brew Moon Restaurant & Microbrewery (established 1994)
    115 Stuart St. (Theatre District), Boston
    (617) 523-6467
    Brew Moon was voted Best of Boston/Best Brewpub by *Boston
    Magazine;* voted one of the Top New Restaurants by *Bon Appetit,*
    and awarded a Gold Medal at the 1996 Great American Beer
    Festival. It's located in the State Transportation Building and easily
    accessible by the T or by car.
    Types of brew: 5 regulars, 2–3 seasonal
    Food style: creative contemporary cuisine

4. Commonwealth Brewing Co. Ltd. (established 1986)
    138 Portland St. (West Side), Boston
    (617) 523-8383
    This well-established brewpub contains antiques from the Original
    Bass Brewery.
    Types of brew: 9 regulars, 1 seasonal
    Food style: American

5. Fort Hill Brew House (established 1996)
    125 Broad St. (Financial District), Boston
    (617) 695-9700
    Located in a renovated barn and factory.
    Types of brew: 6 regulars
    Food style: American

6. Brew Moon Restaurant & Microbrewery (established 1996)
    50 Church St. (Harvard Square), Cambridge
    (617) 523-6467
    This brewpub opened following the success of the Brew Moon in
    Boston. The pub has a "historically influenced interior design."
    which means everything looks old, but is really brand new.
    Types of brew: 5 regulars, 2–3 seasonal
    Food style: Creative contemporary cuisine

7. Cambridge Brewing Co. (established 1989)
   1 Kendall Square, Building 100 (Near MIT), Cambridge
   (617) 494-1994
   Types of brew: 4 regulars, 1–2 seasonal
   Food style: varies

8. John Harvard's Brew House (established 1992)
   33 Dunster Street (Harvard Square), Cambridge
   (617) 868-3585
   In this brewpub, you'll find what are purported to be William
   Shakespeare's Homebrew Recipes on display.
   Types of brew: 5 regulars, 1–3 seasonal
   Food style: American

Boston University School of Medicine

Harvard Medical School

Tufts University School of Medicine

Manhattan

1. A. J. Gordon's Brewing Co. (established 1996)
   212 W. 79th Street (Upper West Side)
   (212) 579-9777
   Types of brew: 4 regulars, 1 seasonal
   Food style: varied, with great specials

2. Carnegie Hill Brewing (established 1995)
   1600 Third Avenue (Upper East Side)
   (212) 369-0808
   Offers Direct TV with sports on an eight-foot screen and 11 other
   TVs sprinkled all through the joint. Fireplace in the lower room.
   Types of brew: 3 regulars, 2 seasonal
   Food style: American

3. Chelsea Brewing Co. (established 1996)
   Pier 59, Chelsea Piers (West side)
   (212) 336-6440

Near the fantastic Chelsea Sports Complex. Get lubricated and try climbing the 60-foot high, rock-climbing practice wall in the health club.
Types of brew: 4 regulars, 2 seasonal
Food style: American/Italian

4. Commonwealth Brewing Co. (established 1996)
   35 W. 48th Street (Midtown)
   Rockefeller Plaza
   (212) 977-2269
   This brewpub is an invasion of New York City by Boston's Commonwealth Brewery.
   Types of brew: 5 regulars, 1 seasonal
   Food style: Varied international

5. Hansen Times Square Brewery Restaurant (established 1996)
   160 West 42nd St. (Times Square)
   Broadway
   (212) 398-1234
   Offers authentic German-style brews in the inauthentic Disneyland atmosphere of the new Times Square. Not much character anymore, but the streets are clean.
   Types of brew: 3 regulars, 1 seasonal
   Food style: Varied

6. Heartland Brewery (established 1995)
   35 Union Square West (Greenwich Village)
   (212) 645-3400
   Located in historical Union Square District. It has hand-painted murals on the old, turn-of-the-century brick walls and canvas inlaid in its 40-foot back bar. Voted New York's best brewpub by *New York Magazine* and New York *Press*.
   Types of brew: 5 regulars, 3 seasonal
   Food style: American

7. Highlander Brewery (established 1996)
    190 Third Ave. (Gramercy Park)
    (212) 979-7268
    An American Bar & Grill with Scottish traditional flavor. Former
    site of Cheffield's German Beer Hall.
    Types of brew: 3 regulars

8. Typhoon Brewery (established 1996)
    22 East 54th St. (Midtown)
    (212) 754-9006
    Types of brew: 4 regulars
    Food style: Traditional Thai

9. West Side Brewing Co. (established 1993)
    340 Amsterdam Ave. (Upper West Side)
    (212) 721-2161
    Types of brew: 4 regulars
    Food style: American

10. Yorkville Brewery & Tavern (established 1994)
    1359 First Ave. (Upper East Side)
    (212) 517-2739
    Types of brew: 3 regulars, 2 seasonals
    Food style: American

11. Zip City Brewing Co. (established 1991)
    3 West 18th St. (Flatiron District)
    (212) 366-6333
    This brewpub was installed in the former home of National
    Temperance Society from the late 1800s. That's cheeky.
    Types of brew: 3 rotating varieties
    Food style: upscale pub fare

Yeshiva University, Albert Einstein College of Medicine, Bronx

Columbia University College of Physicians and Surgeons

Cornell University Medical College

Mount Sinai School of Medicine of the City University of New York

New York University School of Medicine

New York Medical College, Valhalla

SUNY Health Science Center at Brooklyn College of Medicine

Chicago

This is an industrial city, so both of these microbreweries are located in abandoned factories. It is an ambiance of sorts.

1. Goose Island Brewing Co. (established 1988)
   1800 North Clybourn
   (312) 915-0071
   Types of brew: 2 regulars, 6 seasonal
   Food style: American

2. River West Brewing Company (established 1996)
   925 W. Chicago Ave.
   Types of brew: 8 regulars, 6 seasonal

University of Chicago, Pritzker School of Medicine

Finch University of Health Sciences, Chicago Medical School

University of Illinois College of Medicine

Loyola University, Chicago Stritch School of Medicine

Northwestern University Medical School

Rush Medical College of Rush University

Cleveland

1. Great Lakes Brewing Co. (established 1988)
   2516 Market Street
   (216) 771-4404
   Located in an historic building in the Ohio City area.
   Types of brew: 3 regulars, 3 seasonals
   Food style: American Bistro

2. Rock Bottom Brewery (established 1995)
2000 Sycamore St. (West Bank of the Flats, Downtown)
(216) 623-1555
Related through ownership to Denver's Rock Bottom Brewery.
Types of brew: 7 regulars
Food style: varied with Southwest flavor

3. Firehouse Brewery
3216 Silsby Road, Cleveland Heights
(216) 932-2739
Brewpub located in landmark 1931 Tudor-style firehouse.
Types of brew: 4 regulars, 2 seasonal
Food style: varied from pub fare to fine dining

Case Western Reserve University School of Medicine, Cleveland

Washington, DC and surrounding areas

1. Capitol City Brewing Co. (established 1992)
1100 New York Avenue, Washington, DC
(202) 628-2222
Guided tours of brewery offered.
Types of brew: 2 regulars, 7 seasonal
Food style: American

2. Capitol City Brewing Co., established 1996
2 Massachusetts Avenue NE, Washington, DC
(202) 842-2337
Located in an historic former postal building (sans Uzi-toting mail carriers) also offers an outdoor patio for alfresco dining and drinks.
Types of brew: 6 regulars, 3 seasonals
Food style: American

3. Virginia Brewing Co. (established 1995)
607 King Street, Alexandria, VA
(703) 684-5397
Types of brew: 8 house
Food style: Creole, seafood

4. Bardo Rodeo (established 1993)
   2000 Wilson Boulevard, Arlington, VA
   (703) 527-9399
   This is the largest brewpub in the country, sporting 24 pool tables.
   With that much fun inside, why the fake Southwestern getup? Just
   decoration is the best guess.
   Types of brew: 11 regulars, 2 seasonal
   Food style: Southwestern American

5. Blue 'n Gold Brewing Co.
   3100 Clarendon Blvd.
   Arlington, VA
   (703) 908-4995
   A highly recommended brewpub with New Orleans atmosphere.
   Types of brew: 6 regulars, 4 seasonals
   Food style: French Creole
   A highly recommended brewpub with New Orleans atmosphere.
   Types of brew: 6 regulars, 4 seasonals
   Food style: French creole

George Washington University School of Medicine and Health Sciences

Georgetown University School of Medicine

Howard University College of Medicine

Uniformed Services University of the Health Sciences, Bethesda

Austin, Texas

You're just going to have to drive to have a good time in Texas. There's
no way around it.

1. Bitter End Bistro & Brewery (established 1994)
   311 Colorado (Warehouse Arts District)
   (512) 478-2337
   Types of brew: 5 regulars, 1 seasonal
   Food style: Contemporary American

2. Copper Tank Brewing Co.
    504 Trinity St. (Sixth Street entertainment district)
    (512) 478-8444
    Types of brew: 5 regulars, 1–2 seasonal
    Food style: Various

3. Waterloo Brewing Co. (established 1994)
    401 Guadalupe Street (Sixth Street entertainment district)
    (512) 477-1836
    First brewpub in Austin, TX
    Types of brew: 5 regulars, 2 seasonal
    Food style: American grill

Texas A&M University Health Science Center, College Station

University of Texas Medical School at San Antonio

Seattle, Washington

1. Big Time Brewing Co. (established 1987)
    4133 University Way, N.E. (University District)
    (206) 545-4509
    This brewpub is only one block from University of Washington.
    Types of brew: 3 regulars, 3 seasonal
    Food style: Pub fare

2. California & Alaska St. Brewpub (established 1991)
    4720 California Avenue
    (206) 938-2476
    This is the only brewpub to be found on Seattle's west side.
    Types of brew: 8 regulars, 1 seasonal
    Food style: Pub fare

3. McMenamins Queen Anne (established 1995)
    200 Roy Street
    (206) 285-4722
    Just two blocks from Seattle Center and Key Arena.
    Types of brew: 7 regulars, 5 seasonal
    Food style: Various

    University of Washington School of Medicine

Salt Lake City, Utah

1. Desert Edge Brewery at The Pub (established 1995)
    273 Trolley Square (Downtown)
    (801) 521-8917
    Only brewpub in area that brews traditional lagers.
    Types of brew: 5 regulars, 1 seasonal
    Food style: eclectic American

2. Fuggles Microbrewery (established 1994)
    367 West 200 South
    (801) 521-7446
    Types of brew: 12 regulars, 1 seasonal

3. Squatter's Pub Brewery (established 1988)
    147 West Broadway
    (801) 363-2739
    Salt Lake City's first brewpub.
    Types of brew: 10 regular, 2 seasonal
    Food style: Both traditional and modern pub fare

University of Utah School of Medicine

SCHOOLS NEAR
SOUR MASH BOURBON DISTILLERIES

Bourbon, that distinctly American drink, is distilled only in Tennessee and Kentucky. Jack Daniels is the benchmark by which all the other whiskies are measured. Unique in taste and mellow in its effects, J.D. it is not simply a great drink: to many of its millions of devotees, it is the only drink. The distillery in Lynchburg, Tennessee, is now owned by Brown-Foreman, a conglomerate that produces about 20 various liquors, but the quality of Jack Daniels remains uncompromised.

The distillery tour is well worth taking. Step into the "aging shed," a wooden building about the size of two football fields with barrels stacked two stories high inside. Breathe in the essence of this noble liquor, let it permeate your pores, then walk back out into the sunshine—a religious experience. Jack Daniels recently introduced their first new whiskey in over a hundred years in an attempt to jump into the growing market for single barrel bourbons—Gentleman Jack. It is a superb sipping whiskey, even superior to Jack Daniel's Black (which is saying a lot). At about $25 a bottle, it's a bargain.

East Tennessee State University College of Medicine, Johnson City

Meharry Medical College School of Medicine, Nashville

Vanderbilt University School of Medicine, Nashville

University of Tennessee College of Medicine, Memphis

The 200-year-old Jim Beam distillery claims a membership of 30,000 in its Jim Beam fan club, known as "The Kentucky Circle." That's nice—but of greater interest is its specialty sour mash whiskey priced at about $25 a fifth. Better yet is a group of what the company calls single-barrel whiskies priced in the $30–$50 range under names like Bakers, Brookers, Basil Hayden, and Knob Creek. All are excellent. Barton's Distillers of Clermont, Kentucky, also produce a fine single barrel along with their Kentucky Tavern and Ten High brands.

Bardstown, Kentucky is the home of Heaven Hill, a rather undistinguished bourbon. However, the company also produces Evan Williams, which is quite good, and moderately priced.

Wild Turkey is distilled to its full 101-proof strength in Lawrenceville, Kentucky. Now the company is marketing a new variety, Rare Breed. Not a single-barrel bourbon, Rare Breed is a blend of different barrels of different ages to create a heavy but effective bourbon.

With everyone jumping on the bourbon bandwagon, it's no surprise that the Twelve Stone Company in Bardstown, Kentucky, is offering American Biker Bourbon. A portrait of a gentleman riding his hawg adorns the label. This picture—and the fact that the price is only about $13 a bottle—are all that recommends this drink. Don't offer it to any self-respecting biker—he or she might bust the bottle over your gourd. How could they presume to challenge the likes of Blanton's, distilled by the Sazerac Company in Frankfort, Kentucky? Sure, Blanton's single-barrel sells for three times as much as American Biker, but it's worth it.

University of Kentucky College of Medicine, Lexington

University of Louisville School of Medicine, Louisville

IN WINE COUNTRY

If you count yourself a connoisseur of America's increasingly well-accepted home-grown wines and world class vintners, you might want to consider a school near the source of your favorite wine region. There are currently wine-producing vineyards in about 20 states. The following list includes the schools in the very best of Wine Country.

California

The Napa Valley

The Napa Valley, less than a two-hours' drive north from San Francisco, is about 3 or 4 miles wide in the south and extends north for 30 miles, narrowing down to less than a mile at the foot of Mt. St. Helena. More than 80 percent of Napa's workable land is under vine. But it is the quality, not the quantity, of the grapes that makes this region distinctive. In the 1960s, Napa began challenging European wine supremacy. Today, some of the best wines in the world come from this region. Here are the schools within striking distance:

University of California School of Medicine, San Francisco

Stanford University School of Medicine, Stanford

The Central Valley

About 90 percent of all the wine made in the America comes from California. Eighty percent of all California wines come from the Central Valley, stretching from Sacramento in the north to Bakersfield in the south. Here you will find the enormous Gallo Winery (with a 175-million gallon capacity, the largest in the world), and the University of California at Davis, the nation's leading wine school. The other schools in this large neighborhood include:

University of California School of Medicine, Davis

The Pacific Northwest

Oregon, Washington, and Idaho

Famous for light, "Northern European" style wines best grown in cool climate vineyards, this area has carved itself a distinctive niche in the wine market. In Oregon, the best vineyards lie near the coastal regions around Portland. In Washington, the vintners have chosen Seattle and the Yakima Valley in the southeastern region of the state. The western regions of Idaho by the Snake River are also coming under successful cultivation.

Oregon Health Sciences University School of Medicine, Portland

University of Washington School of Medicine, Seattle

New York State

Upstate and the Finger Lakes Region

New York makes more "bottle fermented" sparkling wine than California. New York's lambrusca grape wine country lies in the vicinity of Buffalo and to the southeast, in the center of the state. The scenic Finger Lakes region provides some great cabernets, comfortable bed and breakfasts and The Bully Hill Winery—one of the finest in the state.

University of Rochester School of Medicine and Dentistry

SUNY at Buffalo School of Medicine and Biomedical Sciences

SUNY Health Science Center at Syracuse College of Medicine

Albany Medical College, Albany

Long Island, NY

Long Island is developing an interesting wine-growing district on its eastern extremity. The relatively temperate climate has begun to produce award-winning Sauvignon, Chardonnay, and dry Cabernet wines. The wine growing district is in the Bridgehampton and North Fork areas, about two hours away from New York City by car, if the Long Island Expressway doesn't happen to be transformed into a total parking lot the day you choose for an outing.

Yeshiva University, Albert Einstein College of Medicine, Bronx

Columbia University College of Physicians and Surgeons

Cornell University Medical College

Mount Sinai School of Medicine of the City University of New York

New York University School of Medicine

New York Medical College, Valhalla

SUNY Health Science Center at Brooklyn College of Medicine

SUNY Stony Brook School of Medicine Health Sciences Center

New York Institute of Technology College of Osteopathic Medicine, Old Westbury

Arkansas

The Altus Region

It ain't just moonshine coming out of the Ozarks anymore. Besides the north-central area of the state, the Altus Region at the Arkansas-Missouri-Oklahoma border was designated an officially controlled wine region in the mid 1980s. Actually, the area has been producing good wine ever since it was settled by Swiss immigrants in the 1870s. Here are the schools near what might become the next "sleeper" district of wine production.

University of Arkansas for Medical Sciences College of Medicine, Little Rock

University of Oklahoma College of Medicine, Oklahoma City

NEAR GREAT TENNIS

Queens, New York

Huh? Well, Queens is the New York City borough in which resides the Forest Hills Tennis Stadium, home each August and September to the U.S. Open. If you can afford the tickets, you can munch $5 hot dogs while watching the greatest tennis players in the world compete.

Yeshiva University, Albert Einstein College of Medicine, Bronx

Columbia University College of Physicians and Surgeons

Cornell University Medical College

Mount Sinai School of Medicine of the City University of New York

New York University School of Medicine

New York Medical College, Valhalla

SUNY Health Science Center at Brooklyn College of Medicine

SUNY Stony Brook School of Medicine Health Sciences Center

New York Institute of Technology College of Osteopathic Medicine, Old Westbury

Boston, Massachusetts area

Venerable Longwood, near Boston, hosted the U.S. Doubles Championships between the 1920s and 1940s. It is still one of the premier tennis clubs in America today.

Boston University School of Medicine

Harvard Medical School, Cambridge

Tufts University School of Medicine

University of Massachusetts School of Medicine, Worcester

Newport, Rhode Island

The beautiful Newport Casino, designed by Stanford White, is the Mecca of American tennis. The casino houses the Tennis Hall of Fame and was the site of the first U.S. Open Tennis championships in 1881.

Brown University School of Medicine, Providence

Sea Bright, New Jersey

This lovely city on the Jersey Shore is the traditional American shrine for grass-court devotees. The old Eastern grass court circuit held their greatest amateur tournaments here and in the city of Orange between the 1920s and 1940s.

University of Medicine and Dentistry of New Jersey, Newark

University of Medicine and Dentistry of New Jersey, Piscataway

Los Angeles, California

This city not only produced Ellsworth Vines and Ellis Marble, but it is also the place where the incomparable Bill Tilden spent his last years making tennis a celebrity sport through his friendships with Charlie Chaplin and many other Hollywood stars. L.A. remains the epicenter of West Coast tennis.

UCLA School of Medicine, Los Angeles

University of Southern California School of Medicine, Los Angeles

Indianapolis, Indiana

Thanks to its being the home of U.S. Tennis Association bigshot Stan Molless, Indianapolis hosts an important indoor tournament and offers tennis facilities and fervor equal to any tennis mad area in the country.

Indiana University School of Medicine

Philadelphia, Pennsylvania, and Jacksonville, Florida

American women's tennis was virtually born at Philadelphia's Belmont Cricket Club in the late 1880s. One of the most prestigious and pleasant tournaments on the Women's tour is the Bausch & Lomb Championship held each spring at the Amelia Island Plantation in Northeast Florida on the beach, not far from Jacksonville. Hear Monica Seles squeeze out her famous two-toned grunt with every backhand as she fights for her share of $450,000 in prize money.

Thomas Jefferson University, Jefferson Medical College, Philadelphia

Medical College of Pennsylvania and Hahnemann University School of Medicine, Philadelphia

University of Pennsylvania School of Medicine, Philadelphia

Temple University School of Medicine, Philadelphia

Philadelphia College of Osteopathic Medicine, Philadelphia

University of Florida School of Medicine, Gainesville

NEAR GREAT BASEBALL

Tampa and St. Petersburg, Florida

The majority of major league teams spend much of February and March each year around the Tampa–St. Pete area for spring training. Get a look at the coming season firsthand, long before it starts in earnest. You can't beat the weather either.

University of South Florida College of Medicine, Tampa

Savannah, Georgia

This old seaport town happens to be home to the AA Savannah Cardinals. Sit close to the field at their cozy ballpark and catch the future stars before they start charging $50 apiece for their autographs.

Emory University School of Medicine, Atlanta

Morehouse School of Medicine, Atlanta

Medical College of Georgia School of Medicine, Augusta

Mercer University School of Medicine, Macon

Phoenix, Arizona

Like southern Florida, Phoenix is also a big spring training camp for major league teams, only minus the ocean. But in the hot, dry air, you'll see plenty of 500-foot home runs.

University of Arizona College of Medicine, Tucson

Midwestern University Arizona College of Osteopathic Medicine, Glendale

Boston, Massachusetts area

Suffer along with Boston fans trying to overcome the "Babe Ruth Curse." For Red Sox rooters, baseball has transcended sport to become a religion. One of the truly great baseball towns.

Boston University School of Medicine

Harvard Medical School, Cambridge

Tufts University School of Medicine

University of Massachusetts School of Medicine, Worcester

Chicago, Illinois

In the Windy City, you have the National League equivalent of the Red Sox: the Cubs. They're perennial bridesmaids and never the brides, but boy, do they have some fanatical fans. And if the Cubs aren't doing well, there's always the White Sox.

University of Chicago, Pritzker School of Medicine

Finch University of Health Sciences, Chicago Medical School

University of Illinois College of Medicine

Loyola University, Chicago Stritch School of Medicine

Northwestern University Medical School

Rush Medical College of Rush University

Cooperstown, New York

Buried in the woods about 75 miles from Albany, easily accessible only by helicopter, is the Baseball Hall of Fame. Baseball was no more invented here than it was in Moscow. But the Hall of Fame is an incredible treasure trove of the game's history and artifacts. The baseball library is incomparable.

University of Rochester School of Medicine and Dentistry

SUNY at Buffalo School of Medicine and Biomedical Sciences

SUNY Health Science Center at Syracuse College of Medicine

Albany Medical College, Albany

Philadelphia, Pennsylvania

You will find the most critical baseball fans on Earth in the City of Brotherly Love. Here they not only booed Mike Schmidt, they'd boo anybody. These rabid but knowledgeable fans offer little love to those who can't play the game (and not much more to those who can).

Thomas Jefferson University, Jefferson Medical College, Philadelphia

Medical College of Pennsylvania and Hahnemann University School of Medicine, Philadelphia

University of Pennsylvania School of Medicine, Philadelphia

Temple University School of Medicine, Philadelphia

Philadelphia College of Osteopathic Medicine, Philadelphia

New York, New York

Come see George Steinbrenner's Yankees and the once-again dipsy-doodle Mets. Watch as players who starred with other teams around the nation crumble beneath the city's inexorable media microscope. And here's one for purists only: In the early 1840s, Alexander Cartwright initiated the first organized baseball team, the Knickerbockers, in New York City. The players—mostly firemen from different parts of town—practiced around the neighborhood now known as Murray Hill. In fact, take a pick and shovel up to the empty lot at 30th Street and Lexington Avenue and dig for baseball artifacts. Sell 'em and pay for your tuition.

Columbia University College of Physicians and Surgeons

Cornell University Medical College

Mount Sinai School of Medicine of the City University of New York

New York University School of Medicine

The Bay Area, California

You risk frostbite at the Giants' windswept, foggy 3Com Park (still known as Candlestick Park, or The Stick, to those who love the place), or dying of loneliness watching the Athletics across the bay in Oakland. But at least you're in San Francisco.

University of San Francisco

University of California School of Medicine, San Francisco

Baltimore, Maryland

Unlike the ugly, inhuman, and inhumane structures erected to house baseball in other cities, the Orioles' Camden Yards has integrity and charm. This is a class-act franchise—and the crab cakes are good, too.

Johns Hopkins School of Medicine

University of Maryland School of Medicine

Uniformed Services University of the Health Sciences, Bethesda

Denver, Colorado

Join the baseball frenzy that has seen Colorado set astounding attendance records every year since the inception of their team. And when the Rockies aren't playing, there's the Rockies—the mountains that is. The beautiful foothills begin about 20 minutes away, outside Boulder.

University of Colorado School of Medicine

Los Angeles, California

Leave the game at Dodger Stadium in the seventh inning (like everyone else does) and drive over to Anaheim to watch the Angels. Nothing beats a two-team town.

UCLA School of Medicine, Los Angeles

University of Southern California School of Medicine, Los Angeles

Buffalo, New York

Buffalo? Yeah, Buffalo, home of the most successful minor-league franchise in the country. With the increasingly prima donna behavior of major leaguers, minor-league baseball has skyrocketed in popularity, and Buffalo is a bastion of the sport the way it ought to be.

SUNY at Buffalo School of Medicine and Biomedical Sciences

Arlington, Texas

Think Texas is football country? Well, you're right—but they support their Rangers, and many of the experts have a sneaky feeling that this will be Texas's first championship baseball team.

University of Texas Southwestern Medical Center at Dallas

University of North Texas Health Science Center College of Osteopathic Medicine, Fort Worth

NEAR GREAT HORSE RACING

Louisville, Kentucky

Not only is Louisville home to the first and brightest star in the triple crown, the Kentucky Derby, the state's bluegrass country raises many of the best thoroughbreds in the world.

University of Kentucky College of Medicine, Lexington

University of Louisville School of Medicine

Baltimore, Maryland

Like Kentucky, Maryland is horse-friendly. Pimlico racetrack hosts the Preakness Stakes, second leg of the triple crown. And Maryland's horse farms are among the best.

Johns Hopkins School of Medicine

University of Maryland School of Medicine

New York, New York

If you love to watch the ponies run in circles, there is no other place quite like New York. Besides hosting the third leg of the triple crown, the Belmont Stakes, at Belmont Park, the Big Apple offers adjacent Aqueduct Racetrack with a quality card for the entire winter. But be warned. If you're thinking of paying your tuition by betting against the locals, think again—New York horse bettors are among the meanest and savviest anywhere. There are few underlays (good, high-odds horses that haven't been discovered by every bettor at the track) here.

Yeshiva University, Albert Einstein College of Medicine, Bronx

Columbia University College of Physicians and Surgeons

Cornell University Medical College

Mount Sinai School of Medicine of the City University of New York

New York University School of Medicine

New York Medical College, Valhalla

SUNY Health Science Center at Brooklyn College of Medicine

Saratoga Springs, New York

This quiet, historical town—site of a famous Revolutionary War battle—wakes up every August as the horsy contingent of high society flies into town from all over the world to participate in Saratoga's summer meet and yearling auction. But it is also known as "the graveyard of favorites" because it rains here nearly every afternoon—no benefit to handicapping.

University of Rochester School of Medicine and Dentistry

SUNY at Buffalo School of Medicine and Biomedical Sciences

SUNY Health Science Center at Syracuse College of Medicine

Albany Medical College, Albany

Oceanside, New Jersey

While there are plenty of city slickers attending the summer meet at Monmouth Park near the Jersey shore, you can still find underlays at Monmouth and at the relatively nearby Philadelphia Park.

University of Medicine and Dentistry of New Jersey, Newark

University of Medicine and Dentistry of New Jersey, Piscataway

Thomas Jefferson University, Jefferson Medical College, Philadelphia

Medical College of Pennsylvania and Hahnemann University School of Medicine, Philadelphia

University of Pennsylvania School of Medicine, Philadelphia

Temple University School of Medicine, Philadelphia

Philadelphia College of Osteopathic Medicine, Philadelphia

Gulfstream and Hialeah, Florida

Thanks to the influx of wiseguy New Yorkers, it's no bargain trying to outthink the locals during winter racing at these two south Florida tracks. But then again, it's January—and at least you're in Florida.

University of Miami School of Medicine, Miami

Nova Southeastern University College of Osteopathic Medicine, North Miami Beach

Santa Anita, California

As the jewel of California tracks, you will see the best of West Coast racing here but with the problems inherent in betting against a knowledgeable horse crowd. Angeleno railbirds are as tough as they come.

University of California College of Medicine, Irvine

UCLA School of Medicine, Los Angeles

University of Southern California School of Medicine, Los Angeles

Loma Linda University School of Medicine, Loma Linda

Western University of Health Sciences College of Osteopathic Medicine of the Pacific, Pomona

Louisiana Downs, Louisiana

Though adjacent to New Orleans and therefore prey to the city's resident sharks, and home of the prestigious Louisiana Derby, this track offers opportunities for the sophisticated bettor who can size up a horse and read between the lines of the racing form.

Louisiana State University School of Medicine in New Orleans

Tulane University School of Medicine, New Orleans

NEAR GREAT FOOTBALL

Green Bay, Wisconsin

This is the number one pick for football fans, not because Green Bay won its first Super Bowl in 30 years in 1997, and not for the immortal Vince Lombardi and his teams of the 1960s, but because Packer fans eat, sleep, live, and die by their community-owned team, regardless of how it fares in the standings. Forget about Dallas and "America's Team." Look to the dairyland and "The People's Team."

Medical College of Wisconsin, Milwaukee

University of Wisconsin Medical School, Madison

Lincoln, Nebraska

Why would anyone want to settle here, adjacent to the High Plains notorious for having the coldest winters and hottest summers in the continental 48? The University of Nebraska Cornhuskers, for starters— the college football powerhouse of the '90s.

University of Nebraska College of Medicine

Creighton University School of Medicine

Canton, Ohio

This city gave birth to the legendary Canton Bulldogs, organized in 1905, when all players played both offense and defense—without helmets. Now Canton is the home of the Pro Football Hall of Fame.

Case Western Reserve University School of Medicine, Cleveland

University of Cincinnati College of Medicine

Medical College of Ohio, Toledo

Northeatern Ohio Universities College of Medicine, Rootsville

Ohio State University College of Medicine, Columbus

Wright State University School of Medicine, Dayton

Jacksonville, Florida

The Bold New City of the South, they call themselves, but Jacksonville was on no one's map until the astounding Jaguars made it to the conference finals in just their second season of existence.

University of Florida College of Medicine, Gainesville

Charlotte, North Carolina

Like the Jaguars, the Carolina Panthers amazed the football world by achieving a first-rate franchise in just their second year. The fans here have years of roaring for the great regional college football teams under their belts. This is not a football town for those with delicate systems.

Bowman Gray School of Medicine of Wake Forest University, Winston-Salem

Duke University School of Medicine, Durham

University of North Carolina at Chapel Hill School of Medicine

East Carolina University School of Medicine, Greenville

Dallas, Texas

Angering the rest of the country by arrogantly declaring themselves "America's Team," the Cowboys are now the prime example of American professional athletes run amok. Still, this is the most successful pro football franchise over the past 30 years, and you can bet they'll be back.

University of Texas Southwestern Medical Center at Dallas

University of North Texas Health Science Center College of Osteopathic Medicine, Fort Worth

Notre Dame, Indiana

While the Fighting Irish have slipped in recent years, this most historically glorious of football schools now houses the College Football Hall of Fame.

Indiana University School of Medicine, Indianapolis

NEAR GREAT HOCKEY

The New York Metropolitan Area

There are three NHL teams within a slap shot of each other: the New Jersey Devils, the New York Rangers, and the New York Islanders. What's more, in the Rangers' Wayne Gretzky you can see the all-time leading scorer, the best playmaker in hockey history, and perhaps the greatest player ever to take to the ice.

Yeshiva University, Albert Einstein College of Medicine, Bronx

Columbia University College of Physicians and Surgeons

Cornell University Medical College

Mount Sinai School of Medicine of the City University of New York

New York University School of Medicine

New York Medical College, Valhalla

SUNY Health Science Center at Brooklyn College of Medicine

SUNY Stony Brook School of Medicine Health Sciences Center

New York Institute of Technology College of Osteopathic Medicine, Old Westbury

University of Medicine and Dentistry of New Jersey, Newark

University of Medicine and Dentistry of New Jersey, Piscataway

Detroit, Michigan

For many years, the Red Wings were led by the immortal Gordie Howe, widely considered one of the greatest players in the history of the game. Now, the Red Wings' leader is the brilliant Sergei Fedorov and his Russian teammates—the wave of the future in the NHL. In 1972, 94 percent of NHL players were Canadian. Today, the figure is 61 percent. Many of the non-Canadian players are American, but most of the best are European, specifically, Russian. Given the size of Russia and the lack of opportunity there, the trend is likely to continue. These Ivans can play.

Wayne State University School of Medicine

Pittsburgh, Pennsylvania

The Penguins are blessed with the best one-two goal scoring punch in the NHL: the great Mario Lemieux (heir to Gretzky), and Jaromir Jagr.

Pennsylvania State University College of Medicine, Hershey

University of Pittsburgh School of Medicine

Lake Erie College of Osteopathic Medicine, Erie

Denver, Colorado

The Avalanche is a new franchise that has reached the pinnacle of success in a fraction of the time that it previously took a championship team to build up steam. Colorado, a young, hard-checking team with plenty of depth, is likely to stay at the top.

University of Colorado School of Medicine

Miami, Florida

The only other ice these people see besides the hockey rink is in their drinks, but The Florida Panthers are another young-but-poised squad that plays strong on the road as well as at home. A team of the future.

University of Miami School of Medicine, Miami

Nova Southeastern University College of Osteopathic Medicine, North Miami Beach

Philadelphia, Pennsylvania

In years past, the Flyers were decried as a dirty-playing goon squad. They were also a darn good team. Now, led by Eric Lindros, they're ba-aaack. Just when you thought it was safe to go back on the ice.

Thomas Jefferson University, Jefferson Medical College, Philadelphia

Medical College of Pennsylvania and Hahnemann University School of Medicine, Philadelphia

University of Pennsylvania School of Medicine, Philadelphia

Temple University School of Medicine, Philadelphia

Philadelphia College of Osteopathic Medicine, Philadelphia

NEAR LEGALIZED GAMBLING

Atlantic City, New Jersey

The new Sodom and Gomorrah by the sea, it is considerably smaller than Las Vegas in terms of hotel rooms and total visitors, but outgrosses its Nevada counterpart in money wagered. With business going so well, perks and "comps" in Atlantic City casinos have diminished for the average visitor. These are reserved for the high rollers (read: proven suckers).

University of Medicine and Dentistry of New Jersey, Newark

University of Medicine and Dentistry of New Jersey, Piscataway

Nevada

Having legalized gambling in 1931, the casino business in Las Vegas and Reno is the most sophisticated in the nation, perhaps the world. Las Vegas is a city with slot machines in public restrooms. There are literally hundreds of places where you can gamble. Because of fierce competition, there are many perks, such as cheap or free food and lodging—if you can prove you're not a local. More importantly for the serious player, the house's take on slots and other rules can vary from casino to casino. Pay attention.

University of Nevada School of Medicine, Reno

Foxwood, Connecticut

The American Indian has finally exacted his revenge on the white man in the form of the reservation casino. None is more successful than the Foxwood casino in west-central Connecticut. How successful? In July 1996, Foxwood had $849 million wagered in their slot machines alone. Rooms average $175 each. So bring your wampum.

University of Connecticut School of Medicine, Farmington

Yale University School of Medicine, New Haven

Iowa

In 1989 Iowa approved riverboat gambling along the Mississippi River in Sioux City and Dubuque. Moreover, there is slot machine gambling at three Iowa racetracks, Prairie Meadows, Bluff Run, and Dubuque.

University of Iowa College of Medicine, Iowa City

University of Osteopathic Medicine and Health Sciences, Des Moines

Illinois

There are currently nine riverboat gambling casinos on the state's waterways. Areas excluded from the 1990 legalization were Lake Michigan and Cook County (Chicago). The principal locations for gambling are Joliet, Rock Island, and Alton.

Southern Illinois University School of Medicine, Springfield

South Dakota

In 1988, casino gambling in a limited form was legalized in Deadwood, South Dakota. Only poker, blackjack, and slot machines could be played, with wagers limited to $5. To the credit of the local voters, an attempt to raise the betting limit to $100 was defeated in a state referendum.

University of South Dakota School of Medicine, Vermillion

Missouri

Following the lead of neighboring Iowa, Missouri approved riverboat gambling in 1992. There are currently six floating casinos in St. Joseph and St. Charles.

St. Louis University Health Sciences Center

Washington University School of Medicine, St. Louis

University of Missouri, Columbia School of Medicine

University of Missouri, Kansas City School of Medicine

University of Health Sciences College of Osteopathic Medicine, Kansas City

Kirksville College of Osteopathic Medicine, Kirksville

Indiana

The Hoosiers cut themselves a piece of the gambling pie in 1993, allowing riverboat gambling in several locations. It's a relatively small industry: There are only 243 gaming tables in the whole state.

Indiana University School of Medicine, Indianapolis

Kansas

The staid folk of this Bible Belt, state-approved gambling on Kansas City riverboats with restricted betting limits. There is also a casino on Indian land 17 miles north of Topeka.

University of Kansas School of Medicine, Kansas City

Minnesota

The Mystic Lake Indian Casino operates on tribal land, attracting bus-loads of daytripping gamblers from as far away as Columbus, Ohio. There is absolutely nothing to distract you from the gaming tables on this reservation.

Mayo Medical School, Rochester

University of Minnesota, Duluth School of Medicine

University of Minnesota Medical School, Minneapolis

Detroit, Michigan

In January 1997, perennially impoverished Detroit decided to try and cash in on legalized gambling by approving "gaming with dice games." Neighboring Windsor, Ontario, had plenty of casino gambling, but the Canadian casinos do not have craps tables. These are banned in Canada because of an English law dating back to 1380, enacted by the King of England to keep his soldiers from blowing their paychecks on backgammon. Detroit is a winner.

Wayne State University School of Medicine

Mississippi

Meandering further down the Big Muddy, we come to Mississippi, which allows riverboat casinos in two locations: in cities along the Mississippi River and on the Gulf coast. There must be something in the water besides mud in the Mighty Mississippi to have inspired so many games of chance in so many otherwise conservative and straight-laced settings.

University of Mississippi School of Medicine, Jackson

Louisiana

In 1992, Louisiana followed the monkey-see, monkey-do tradition of state-sanctioned gambling by approving casinos a year after Mississippi did the same. Currently there are 11 casinos operating in New Orleans, Shreveport, and Baton Rouge.

Louisiana State University School of Medicine in New Orleans

Tulane University School of Medicine, New Orleans

Louisiana State University School of Medicine in Shreveport

Arizona

In the vicinity of Tucson, there is the Desert Diamond Casino, operated by the Tohono O'odham Indians. This is the Old West scenery of John Wayne westerns, cheek by jowl with the lights and buzz of slots and the click of the poker chips.

University of Arizona School of Medicine, Tucson

Midwestern University Arizona College of Osteopathic Medicine, Glendale

California

Sprinkled liberally across the state, there are 13,000 electronic slot machines operating on various Indian reservations, including the Crystal Mountain Casino outside of Sacramento. The nearby state legislators are trying to close the place down. Stay tuned.

University of California School of Medicine, Davis

NEAR GREAT BASKETBALL

Chicago

Combine the incomparable Michael Jordan, the merely excellent Scottie Pippin, and the rebounding machine that is Dennis Rodman, and you have the Chicago Bulls, a team with depth in every direction. Jordan and Pippin are no longer spring chickens, and Rodman is in constant danger of self-destruction. Sooner or later, they will stop dominating the NBA. But don't hold your breath waiting.

University of Chicago, Pritzker School of Medicine

Finch University of Health Sciences, Chicago Medical School

University of Illinois College of Medicine

Loyola University, Chicago Stritch School of Medicine

Northwestern University Medical School

Rush Medical College of Rush University

Miami

Despite his Armani suits, slicked-back hair, avarice, and ego, Pat Riley can coach. Without using a single player drafted by the team, he has fashioned the Heat into a top-flight contender. Get out of the kitchen.

University of Miami School of Medicine, Miami

Nova Southeastern University College of Osteopathic Medicine, North Miami Beach

Washington, DC

The Washington Wizards (formerly known as the Bullets) continue to misfire. But John Thompson's Georgetown Hoyas (alma mater of Patrick Ewing and Alonzo Mourning), remains a college powerhouse.

George Washington University School of Medicine and Health Sciences

Georgetown University School of Medicine

Howard University College of Medicine

Uniformed Services University of the Health Sciences, Bethesda

Los Angeles

See the Hollywood stars ensconced in those TV camera-friendly court-side seats! See the 300 pound behemoth, Shaquille O'Neal, brutishly slam dunk his way to an astounding average 25 points per game! He may be a one-trick pony, this Shaq, but he may make the Lakers the next NBA dynasty.

University of Southern California

University of California, Los Angeles

Loyola Marymount University

California State University, Los Angeles

California State University, Long Beach

California State University, Fullerton

Boston

Once proud, now clueless, the Celtics flounder in last place again. Still, there is basketball joy in Beantown thanks to Boston University and Boston College. Both Division I schools play right at the top of their tough conferences. And that includes the female side at Boston College, whose women's basketball team is one of the best in the Big East.

Boston College

University of Boston

Seattle

Thanks to superstars Shawn Kemp and Gary Payton, the Supersonics fly high over the Northwest. Both Kemp and Payton average 20+ points a game, with Kemp among the league leaders in rebounds and Payton likewise in assists. Both should be around long enough to lead Seattle past their usual playoff doldrums into the realm of truly elite NBA teams.

University of Washington school of Medicine, Seattle

Philadelphia

Although the Philadelphia 76'ers are just about eighty-sixed off the NBA map, at least there is Villanova. In a town where the glass is always half empty, the Wildcats have earned raves with their fourth consecutive 20+ win season and by breaking the school record of 91 wins in four seasons.

Thomas Jefferson University, Jefferson Medical College, Philadelphia

Medical College of Pennsylvania and Hahnemann University School of Medicine, Philadelphia

University of Pennsylvania School of Medicine, Philadelphia

Temple University School of Medicine, Philadelphia

Philadelphia College of Osteopathic Medicine, Philadelphia

Connecticut

By capturing the attention and admiration of the country, the women's basketball team at the University of Connecticut was a huge factor in the

recent formation of a women's professional basketball league. It's difficult to say how the pro league will fare, but the Connecticut ladies keep
rolling on.

University of Connecticut School of Medicine, Farmington

Yale University School of Medicine, New Haven

NEAR GREAT GOLF

You may want to pick your school by its accessibility to great courses
and golfing history.

New Haven, Connecticut

The best on-campus golf course of any U.S. medical school:

Yale University School of Medicine

Augusta, Georgia

This small southern town, draped in Spanish moss and honeyed drawls,
is the home of the most prestigious of Professional Golf Association
Tournaments, The Masters, held annually at the Augusta National Golf
Club.

Emory University School of Medicine, Atlanta

Morehouse School of Medicine, Atlanta

Medical College of Georgia School of Medicine, Augusta

Mercer University School of Medicine, Macon

Shinnecock Hills, Long Island

It's one of the most venerable courses in the country, although you'll
probably have to caddy to get on the course at all. Very snobby, very
expensive.

SUNY Stony Brook School of Medicine Health Sciences Center

New York Institute of Technology College of Osteopathic Medicine,
Old Westbury

Yonkers, New York

Yonkers, just north of New York City, is not one of the world's garden spots. But it is where the St. Andrews Golf Course is located (named after the famous Scottish course where golf as we know it was devised). Founded in 1888, St. Andrews Country Club is the oldest American golf club.

New York Medical College, Valhalla

Yeshiva University, Albert Einstein College of Medicine, Bronx

Newport, Rhode Island

Golf was first taken up by American rich folk on summer vacation in Newport in the 1880s. The first U.S. Amateur Tournament took place at the Newport Golf Club in 1895. This is a great place to hang your knickers and spikes.

Brown University School of Medicine, Providence

Pebble Beach, California

Located along the Monterey Peninsula, with some of the most breathtaking Pacific Ocean views on the West Coast as a backdrop, Pebble Beach Golf Club is perhaps the most beautiful and one of the most challenging courses in America today. And even though the course cost its new Japanese owners a lot of yen, you can still play 18 holes here for only $150—not bad for a world-class course.

University of California School of Medicine, San Francisco

Stanford University School of Medicine, Stanford

Fort Worth, Texas

Play the links of the Colonial Country Club and you are walking in the footsteps of perhaps the greatest of all golf legends—Ben Hogan. In fact, Hogan was instrumental in gathering the funding and the original membership for this fantastic course.

University of Texas Southwestern Medical Center at Dallas

University of North Texas Health Science Center College of Osteopathic Medicine, Fort Worth

Los Angeles, California

Not only are there hundreds of golf courses in the L.A. area, this is also Tiger Woods's hometown. Woods is long and straight off the tee, and more accurate than other players on the PGA Tour who are consistently 50 yards shorter on their drives. And look at all the prize money he's piled up in a year. Recommendation: Move to Los Angeles, follow Woods around, breathe the same air, see what happens—maybe his incredible talent will rub off. It could happen.

University of California College of Medicine, Irvine

UCLA School of Medicine, Los Angeles

University of Southern California School of Medicine, Los Angeles

Loma Linda University School of Medicine, Loma Linda

Western University of Health Sciences College of Osteopathic Medicine of the Pacific, Pomona

Bethpage, New York

Of the thousands of public golf courses in America, the five in Bethpage, Long Island—The Red, Yellow, Blue, Green, and the 7,000 yard Black—are among the very best. How good is the Black? Good enough to host the U.S. Open in 2002.

SUNY Health Science Center at Brooklyn College of Medicine

SUNY Stony Brook School of Medicine Health Sciences Center

New York Institute of Technology College of Osteopathic Medicine, Old Westbury

NEAR GREAT STOCK CAR RACING

There may be no sport in the U.S. so like the clash of gladiators as the competition on the NASCAR circuit. If, like many Americans, you have motor oil running in your veins instead of blood, then choose a school from the following list.

Daytona Beach, Florida

The headquarters of NASCAR and host to the crown jewel of the Winston Cup Series, the Daytona 500, this city launches each year's NASCAR race schedule and is also the site of the Pepsi 400 in mid-summer.

University of Florida College of Medicine, Gainesville

Atlanta, Georgia

The Atlanta Speedway hosts the Primestar 500 around Easter and the final race in the Winston Cup series in the fall, the NAPA 500.

Emory University School of Medicine, Atlanta

Morehouse School of Medicine, Atlanta

Medical College of Georgia School of Medicine, Augusta

Mercer University School of Medicine, Macon

Darlington, South Carolina

The circuit moves to Darlington for the TranSouth Financial 400 (What kind of name is that for a stock car race?). And the main event of the circuit on Labor Day is the Mountain Dew 500.

Medical University of South Carolina College of Medicine, Charleston

University of South Carolina School of Medicine, Columbia

Fort Worth, Texas

The Texas Motor Speedway is home of the important Interstate Batteries 500.

University of Texas Southwestern Medical Center at Dallas

University of North Texas Health Science Center College of Osteopathic Medicine, Fort Worth

Bristol, Tennessee

Bristol is the raceway used for the running of the venerable Food City 500 in the early Spring. Then the first night race of the season is the Goody's 500 in August with a starting time of 7:30 PM.

East Tennessee State University College of Medicine, Johnson City

Meharry Medical College School of Medicine, Nashville

Vanderbilt University School of Medicine, Nashville

University of Tennessee College of Medicine, Memphis

Talladega, Alabama

Talladega checks in with the Winston 500 in early April, then hosts the Sears Diehard 500 for the diehard men and machines as the schedule is winding down at the end of the circuit.

University of Alabama School of Medicine, Birmingham

University of Southern Alabama College of Medicine, Mobile

Sonoma and Fontana, California

They'll be saving tires and engines during Sonoma's short three-hour Save Mart 300, and Fontana is the site of the NAPA California 500 in late June.

University of California School of Medicine, Davis

University of California College of Medicine, Irvine

UCLA School of Medicine, Los Angeles

University of Southern California School of Medicine, Los Angeles

University of California School of Medicine, San Diego

University of California School of Medicine, San Francisco

Loma Linda University School of Medicine, Loma Linda

Stanford University School of Medicine, Stanford

Western University of Health Sciences College of Osteopathic Medicine of the Pacific, Pomona

Dover, Delaware

Dover's home to the Miller 500 on June 1, and the MBNA 400 in September.

Johns Hopkins School of Medicine

University of Maryland School of Medicine

Thomas Jefferson University, Jefferson Medical College, Philadelphia

Medical College of Pennsylvania and Hahnemann University School of Medicine, Philadelphia

University of Pennsylvania School of Medicine, Philadelphia

Temple University School of Medicine, Philadelphia

Philadelphia College of Osteopathic Medicine, Philadelphia

University of Medicine and Dentistry of New Jersey, Newark

University of Medicine and Dentistry of New Jersey, Piscataway

Pocono, Pennsylvania

The schedule starts heating up now as the stars, Jeff Gordon, Dale Jarret, Ricky Rudd, Sterling Marlin, Terry Labonte (last year's champ) and "Ironhead" Dale Earnhardt settle into the long groove of summer racing with The Pocono 500.

Thomas Jefferson University, Jefferson Medical College, Philadelphia

Medical College of Pennsylvania and Hahnemann University School of Medicine, Philadelphia

University of Pennsylvania School of Medicine, Philadelphia

Temple University School of Medicine, Philadelphia

Philadelphia College of Osteopathic Medicine, Philadelphia

Pennsylvania State University College of Medicine, Hershey

University of Pittsburgh School of Medicine

Lake Erie College of Osteopathic Medicine, Erie

Brooklyn, Michigan

This is the site of the Miller 400 in June and the ITW Devilbliss 400 in August.

Michigan State University College of Human Medicine, East Lansing

University of Michigan Medical School, Ann Arbor

Wayne State University School of Medicine, Detroit

Loudon, New Hampshire

Loudon replaces North Wilkesboro on the NASCAR circuit with the Jiffy Lube 300, and late in the season, the New Hampshire 300 at the New Hampshire International Raceway.

Dartmouth Medical School

Indianapolis, Indiana

Home of the famous Indianapolis 500 and one of the most important races on the NASCAR schedule, the Brickyard 400 in August.

Indiana University School of Medicine

Watkins Glen, New York

Watkins Glen is the site of the first Formula I Grand Prix of the United States, dating back to 1964. It remains an important Indy Car and stock car circuit track, playing host to many races, including The Bud in the Glen Race in mid-Summer.

University of Rochester School of Medicine and Dentistry

SUNY at Buffalo School of Medicine and Biomedical Sciences

SUNY Health Science Center at Syracuse College of Medicine

Albany Medical College, Albany

Richmond and Martinsville, Virginia

Richmond hosts the Pontiac Excitement 400 early in the season and the Miller 400 in September, one of two night races on the circuit.

Martinsville is the headquarters for the Goody's 500 in the spring. If you show up in Martinsville wearing only your BVDs in late fall, they might make you eat your shorts at the gate of the Hanes 500.

Eastern Virginia Medical School of the Medical College of Hampton Roads, Norfolk

Virginia Commonwealth University Medical College, Richmond

University of Virginia School of Medicine, Charlottesville

West Virginia School of Medicine, Morgantown

West Virginia School of Osteopathic Medicine, Lewis

Marshall University School of Medicine, Huntington

Charlotte and Rockingham, North Carolina

Look to Charlotte for the grueling Coca-Cola 600 early in the season. The labor and management join hands in the UAW-GM Quality 500 in early October. Rockingham hosts the Goodwrench Service Race in the Spring, and the AC-Delco in late October—the brands change, but the tension remains the same.

Bowman Gray School of Medicine of Wake Forest University, Winston-Salem

Duke University School of Medicine, Durham

University of North Carolina at Chapel Hill School of Medicine

East Carolina University School of Medicine, Greenville

Phoenix, Arizona

A recent entrant on the circuit, Phoenix hosts the Dura-Lube 500 in the late fall, the next-to-last race of the season.

University of Arizona College of Medicine, Tucson

Midwestern University Arizona College of Osteopathic Medicine, Glendale

NEAR GREAT MUSEUMS

It takes many years of careful study to gain a true appreciation of great art. However, great art appreciates very quickly—it's a good investment if you know what you're doing. You won't be buying Rubens and Rembrandt with your first Christmas bonus, but you should be knowledgeable enough about art not to snap up a bunch of fake Dali prints on the first excursion into the Art World. So visit a few museums, decide what you like, then snap up something with lasting value.

Atlanta, Georgia

Atlanta's High Museum of Art is a beacon of artistic heritage in the blank canvas of the Deep South.

Emory University School of Medicine, Atlanta

Morehouse School of Medicine, Atlanta

Baltimore, Maryland

No weak sister to neighboring Washington when it comes to fine art, Baltimore offers eight museums, including the noted Baltimore Museum of Art, and it's a short drive to the National collections in the Capitol.

Johns Hopkins School of Medicine

University of Maryland School of Medicine

Boston, Massachusetts area

These days we forget that Boston once was the cultural arbiter for the nation. The vestige of that power remains only in the phrase "Banned in Boston." Boston contains no less than 25 museums, including the internationally renowned Museum of Fine Arts.

Boston University School of Medicine

Harvard Medical School, Cambridge

Tufts University School of Medicine

University of Massachusetts School of Medicine, Worcester

Chicago, Illinois

The Second City in the United States (Los Angeles is still more a concept than a city) claims 19 museums, most notably the Art Institute of Chicago and the Museum of Contemporary Art.

University of Chicago, Pritzker School of Medicine

Finch University of Health Sciences, Chicago Medical School

University of Illinois College of Medicine

Loyola University, Chicago Stritch School of Medicine

Northwestern University Medical School

Rush Medical College of Rush University

Cleveland, Ohio

Cleveland? Yes, Cleveland. Local industrialists have thrown big bucks behind their civic pride over the years, and the residents have a right to be proud of the city's nine museums, particularly The Cleveland Museum of Art.

Case Western Reserve University School of Medicine

Dallas, Texas

You've seen the soap opera reruns, now visit their museums (It won't take nearly as long as it took to find out who shot J.R.—there are only three museums dedicated to the arts in Dallas). If cattle and oil have you all tied up, then at least spend a day at the Dallas Museum of Art.

University of Texas Southwestern Medical Center at Dallas

Detroit, Michigan

Despite its recent woes as undertaker to the automotive industry in America, the city has long had a rich and diverse cultural life. Detroit offers eight museums. The Detroit Institute of the Arts and the Henry Ford Museum are outstanding.

Wayne State University School of Medicine, Detroit

Fort Worth, Texas

Although smaller and living in the shadow of its neighbor, Dallas, Fort Worth has four museums, one more than Dallas. Of national prominence is the Fort Worth Museum of Art.

University of North Texas Health Science Center College of Osteopathic Medicine, Fort Worth

Los Angeles–Long Beach, California

Smog-besotted outside, but culture rich indoors, the Los Angeles basin is home to 33 museums, the greatest of which are the California State University at Long Beach Museum, the J. Paul Getty Museum (perhaps the best endowed cultural institution in the nation), and Los Angeles County Museum of Art.

University of California College of Medicine, Irvine

UCLA School of Medicine, Los Angeles

University of Southern California School of Medicine, Los Angeles

Loma Linda University School of Medicine, Loma Linda

Western University of Health Sciences College of Osteopathic Medicine of the Pacific, Pomona

Minneapolis–St. Paul, Minnesota

Two of the Twin Cities' six museums have achieved international renown: the Minneapolis Institute of Arts and the Minnesota Museum of Art.

Mayo Medical School, Rochester

University of Minnesota, Duluth School of Medicine
University of Minnesota Medical School, Minneapolis

New York, New York

For those of you who haven't been paying attention, New York is the planet's capital in many areas, including museums. Of the 52 museums in Gotham, at least 7 are of world-class stature: American Craft

Museum, Brooklyn Museum, Frick Collection, Metropolitan Museum of Art, Museum of Modern Art, Pierpont Morgan Library and Art Museum, and Solomon Guggenheim Museum.

Yeshiva University, Albert Einstein College of Medicine, Bronx

Columbia University College of Physicians and Surgeons

Cornell University Medical College

Mount Sinai School of Medicine of the City University of New York

New York University School of Medicine

SUNY Health Science Center at Brooklyn College of Medicine

Philadelphia, Pennsylvania

"All things considered," reads the tombstone of Philly native W. C. Fields, "I'd rather be in Philadelphia." The city takes a lot of guff these days on many fronts, but not so much from art lovers. There are 11 museums in Philly, two of which are particularly respected: Pennsylvania Academy of Fine Arts and the Philadelphia Museum of Art.

Thomas Jefferson University, Jefferson Medical College, Philadelphia

Medical College of Pennsylvania and Hahnemann University School of Medicine, Philadelphia

University of Pennsylvania School of Medicine, Philadelphia

Temple University School of Medicine, Philadelphia

Philadelphia College of Osteopathic Medicine, Philadelphia

San Francisco, California

The seventeen museums that grace the Golden Gate are eclectic in nature, like the city itself, including: the Asian Art Museum of San Francisco, the Cartoon Art Museum, the Fine Arts Museum of San Francisco, and the Ansel Adams Center for Photography.

University of California School of Medicine, San Francisco

Tampa-St. Petersburg, Florida

There are nine museums around Tampa Bay, but perhaps the most intriguing is the Salvador Dali Museum. Don't miss the Scarfone Gallery.

University of South Florida College of Medicine

Washington, DC

The capitol's museums rival Paris, Rome, London, and New York, and what's more, the vast majority of them have free admission. This is art for art's sake, and the sake of the people. Of the 30 important museums here, at least eight are as good as any on Earth: Corcoran Gallery of Art, Hirschorn Museum and Sculpture Gallery, National Gallery of Art, National Museum of African Art, National Museum of American Art, National Portrait Galley, Phillips Collection, and The Wilderness Society's Ansel Adams Collection.

George Washington University School of Medicine and Health Sciences

Georgetown University School of Medicine

Howard University College of Medicine

Uniformed Services University of the Health Sciences, Bethesda

NEAR GREAT CLASSICAL MUSIC

Music soothes the savage beast and the savaged grad student. The following cities are standouts—among the top 25 cities in North America—in terms of musically related performing arts: ballet, opera, and classical orchestras. Quantity does not necessarily mean quality musical performance, so the cities have been listed alphabetically.

Atlanta, Georgia

The cultural hub of the South has a ballet company, an opera company, and seven orchestras.

Emory University School of Medicine, Atlanta

Morehouse School of Medicine, Atlanta

Baltimore, Maryland

Baltimore's ballet and opera companies each average 75 dates a year. Its orchestras present over 250 concerts annually.

Johns Hopkins School of Medicine

University of Maryland School of Medicine

Boston, Massachusetts area

One of the top 10 cultural centers in the United States, Boston has two ballet companies, four opera companies, and 23 orchestras.

Boston University School of Medicine

Harvard Medical School, Cambridge

Tufts University School of Medicine

University of Massachusetts School of Medicine, Worcester

Charlotte, North Carolina

Not yet a fully fledged rival to Atlanta, but this rapidly growing city is getting there. An opera company and four orchestras are located here.

Bowman Gray School of Medicine of Wake Forest University, Winston-Salem

Duke University School of Medicine, Durham

University of North Carolina at Chapel Hill School of Medicine

East Carolina University School of Medicine, Greenville

Chicago, Illinois

Chicago offers the musical cornucopia one would expect from a great American city, including a ballet company, nine opera companies, and 27 orchestras.

University of Chicago, Pritzker School of Medicine

Finch University of Health Sciences, Chicago Medical School

University of Illinois College of Medicine

Loyola University, Chicago Stritch School of Medicine

Northwestern University Medical School

Rush Medical College of Rush University

Detroit, Michigan

The metro area's opera and 12 orchestras perform at an average rate of better than one date a day. There are 12 of them here, and an opera company too.

Michigan State University College of Human Medicine, East Lansing

University of Michigan Medical School, Ann Arbor

Wayne State University School of Medicine, Detroit

Los Angeles, California

There are plenty of jokes about tinsel town. Los Angeles, though, is rated second in North America behind New York in terms of classical music by the *Places Rated Almanac*—a high lowbrow kind of burg. Three ballet companies, seven opera companies, and 25 orchestras call this place home.

University of California College of Medicine, Irvine

UCLA School of Medicine, Los Angeles

University of Southern California School of Medicine, Los Angeles

Loma Linda University School of Medicine, Loma Linda

Western University of Health Sciences College of Osteopathic Medicine of the Pacific, Pomona

Milwaukee, Wisconsin

Milwaukee deserves mention for a fine, well rounded musical agenda far out of proportion to its size. It has two ballet companies, three opera companies, and six orchestras.

Medical College of Wisconsin, Milwaukee

University of Wisconsin Medical School, Madison

Minneapolis–St Paul, Minnesota

The nine orchestras in the Twin Cities play a combined total of nearly 500 dates a year. Three opera companies are also based here.

Mayo Medical School, Rochester

University of Minnesota, Duluth School of Medicine

University of Minnesota Medical School, Minneapolis

Newark, New Jersey

In the shadow of the megalithic New York scene, the Garden State centers its musical culture program in Newark with two ballet companies, four opera companies, and 12 orchestras.

University of Medicine and Dentistry of New Jersey, Newark

University of Medicine and Dentistry of New Jersey, Piscataway

New York, New York

New York City is the classical music center of the nation—and of the world too. What are we talking about here? New York's 40 ballet companies, 35 opera companies, and 37 orchestras each schedule over a thousand separate playing dates a year. Moreover, five FM radio stations play over 500 hours of classical music a week.

Yeshiva University, Albert Einstein College of Medicine, Bronx

Columbia University College of Physicians and Surgeons

Cornell University Medical College

Mount Sinai School of Medicine of the City University of New York

New York University School of Medicine

SUNY Health Science Center at Brooklyn College of Medicine

Philadelphia, Pennsylvania

Sixteen symphony orchestras, two ballet companies, and three opera companies are just the tip of the iceberg in this city.

Thomas Jefferson University, Jefferson Medical College, Philadelphia

Medical College of Pennsylvania and Hahnemann University School of Medicine, Philadelphia

University of Pennsylvania School of Medicine, Philadelphia

Temple University School of Medicine, Philadelphia

Philadelphia College of Osteopathic Medicine, Philadelphia

San Francisco, California

Definitely in the top ten American cities in terms of live musical performance, with three ballet companies, three opera companies, and nine orchestras. The classical tradition is yet a further jewel in the Gray Lady's crown.

University of California School of Medicine, San Francisco

San Jose, California

Down the road from San Francisco, this burgeoning, silicon-powered city takes its culture seriously. Three opera companies and four orchestras reside here.

Stanford University School of Medicine

Seattle, Washington

The cultural mecca of the Northwest offers an escape from depression brought on by gray skies and constant drizzle, in the form of two ballet companies, two opera companies, and six orchestras.

University of Washington School of Medicine

St. Louis, Missouri

The local symphony is a world class outfit, playing in a world class hall. St. Louis is another city with a cultural life that far exceeds its size. A ballet company, an opera company, and six orchestras can be found here.

St. Louis University Health Sciences Center

Washington University School of Medicine, St. Louis

Washington, DC

The Wolftrap festival, the Washington Ballet, 21 orchestras, 9 operas, and a ballet company in the metropolitan area make the nation's capitol a wonderful place to listen.

George Washington University School of Medicine and Health Sciences

Georgetown University School of Medicine

Howard University College of Medicine

Uniformed Services University of the Health Sciences, Bethesda

NEAR ROCK AND ROLL LEGENDS

Duluth, Minnesota

Robert Zimmerman was born in this city in 1941 and grew up in Hibbing, a little mining town in the isolated northern reaches of the state. His father ran the local hardware store. In 1960, Robert left home to attend the University of Minnesota, but within a few months he had disappeared off the face of the Earth and was reborn in New York's Greenwich Village as Bob Dylan, folk singer. Dylan has been a protest singer, a rock star, a born-again Christian, a saint to some, and a sellout to others. His songs, from "Blowin' in the Wind" to "All Along the Watchtower" to the more recent novelistic rock ballads like "Tweeter & the Monkeyman" (recorded with The Traveling Wilburys), constitute some of the most powerfully poetic lyrics in popular music. If you're a rebel and a poet, Minnesota's for you.

Mayo Medical School, Rochester

University of Minnesota, Duluth School of Medicine

University of Minnesota Medical School, Minneapolis

Port Arthur, Texas

Lit by the gas flares of the cracking plants, Port Arthur is held together by rust, oil, and humidity. This industrial seaport, strapped onto the

Sabine-Neches Ship Canal, became the birthplace of Janis Joplin on January 19, 1943. Looking around this town, there's no secret about where she got her grit. Janis ran away from home at the age of 17 to Houston and sang in country and western bands, moving on to San Francisco, where she hooked up with Big Brother and the Holding Company in 1966. One year later, she knocked 'em dead at the Monterey Pop Festival with her gut-wrenching rendition of "Ball and Chain." Success came fast and hard. By October 4, 1970, Janis had died of a drug overdose in Hollywood. See what you can do with these roots.

Baylor College of Medicine, Houston

University of Texas Houston Medical School

University of Texas Medical School at Galveston

Freehold, New Jersey

Bruce Springsteen was born in Freehold on September 23, 1949. At the age of 13, he bought himself a guitar after seeing Elvis on television. By the early 1970s, he had formed the E Street Band and soon had a cult following of fans all over the Northeast. National stardom wasn't far behind. With the release of *Born to Run* in 1975 and his first national tour, Bruce truly became The Boss of American Rock and Roll. There is no better working-class love song than "Thunder Road." Don't get too wrapped up in rock and roll, though, or you'll end up a college drop-out like Springsteen.

University of Medicine and Dentistry of New Jersey, Newark

University of Medicine and Dentistry of New Jersey, Piscataway

Memphis, Tennessee

There's only one place to go to school for a fan of Elvis Aron Presley, and that's near Graceland, a shrine to the memory of a man, his music, and his tasteless self-indulgence. Born in Tupelo, Mississippi, in 1935, The King started out as a pauper, the only son of poor sharecroppers who moved to Memphis in 1948. When Elvis was discovered in 1954 by Sam Phillips, the president of Sun Records, he had a high school diploma and was driving a truck. But his swiveling loins and shock of pomaded black hair soon had the sanitized world of American entertainment all shook up. "Heartbreak Hotel," "Hound Dog," "Don't Be Cruel"—his songs hit number one on the charts one after the other and stayed there. Maybe it was the Army, overwhelming fame, or Colonel Tom Parker that ruined the King, but except for a great televised Christmas special in 1968, Elvis ran too fat and out of steam after 1960. His last live performances in Las Vegas were trite and without passion. Elvis retreated behind the gates of Graceland with a band of fawning flunkies, and there he died of an accidental drug overdose in 1977.

University of Tennessee College of Medicine, Memphis

Bay City, Michigan

Madonna Louise Ciccone was born here, near the shores of Lake Huron's Saginaw Bay in 1958. She has passed from the rock and roll scene into legend, a status bestowed on performers who find themselves getting a gazillion dollars for anything they choose to do (no matter what it is), and who have passed over from the "Hey, here I am! Take my picture, take my picture!" phase to the "Why won't they just leave me alone?" state of mind. You won't see Madonna's new baby here, but you might get some insight into "Who's That Girl" behind the bra.

Michigan State University College of Human Medicine, East Lansing

University of Michigan Medical School, Ann Arbor

Augusta, Georgia

The Godfather of Soul burst on the scene in 1956 with his first successful single, "Please, Please, Please," and his influence on soul, rock, rap, and international music has reverberated far beyond his humble beginnings in Augusta, where he was born in 1933. His hits include, "Papa's Got a Brand New Bag," "It's a Man's World," and "Living in America." James Brown is out of jail again and is often spotted in northern Georgia, near his home. If you want to dig into the real roots of rap, talk to the Man. "Mama, come here quick, and bring me that lickin' stick!"

Medical College of Georgia School of Medicine, Augusta

Cleveland, Ohio

In the heart of the nation, the heart of rock beats in perpetuity at the Rock and Roll Hall of Fame and Museum. It took more than ten years of planning, wheedling, and fundraising among the executives and stars of the music industry and the city fathers and captains of industry in Cleveland, but on Labor Day of 1995 the Hall of Fame opened its doors to the public. The museum is sort of like the interior of every Hard Rock Cafe in the world—only more so, and without burgers. The walls are festooned with electric guitars, extravagant outfits, and original manuscripts of famous lyrics written on cocktail napkins and spiral bound notebook paper. Although some rock artists see being inducted into the Hall of Fame as a death knell marking the end of their careers, the museum has meant a rebirth for the blighted Cleveland inner city. I. M. Pei designed the striking building, which is embellished with a huge glass pyramid that houses the Hall of Fame. Now that the induction ceremony and show for new members in the Hall of Fame has moved from New York and L.A. to Cleveland, you might actually see a real rock and roll star in town.

Case Western Reserve University School of Medicine

NEAR GREAT COUNTRY & WESTERN MUSIC

Nashville, Tennessee

The cradle of country music, and home of the Grand Ole Opry, Nashville is still the thriving, thrumming heartbeat of C&W, from the sequined, big band sound to retro cowboy songs. Stay out all night in the clubs lining the recently revitalized main drag downtown, listening to and dancing along with the best that Nashville has to offer. Tour the Opry and pretend you're the late great King of Country Music, Roy Acuff, whose reign on this stage lasted from 1938 to 1992. Visit the Country Music Hall of Fame, stand on Patsy Cline's sidewalk star, and maybe pick up some of the vibes left behind by the happiest girl in the whole U.S.A.

Meharry Medical College School of Medicine

Vanderbilt University School of Medicine

Austin Texas

Stroll down Sixth Street in downtown Austin on a slow night, and you'll hear as much good music as anywhere in America. On the weekends, the town is simply gangbusters with great country & western acts. You could find yourself shaking hands with the late-blooming cult hero and "Zen cowboy," Jimmy Dale Gilmore. Get studio audience tickets for the recording of the PBS show "Austin City Limits."

Texas A&M University Health Science Center, College Station

University of Texas Medical School at San Antonio

Bakersfield, California

Country and western music was stowed in the beat-up baggage of migrant farm workers, who moved to Southern California in their attempt to escape the Dust Bowl in the 1930s. The burg of Bakersfield became the Nashville of the West—without any of the Tennessee city's industry clout. But this is the place that roughed out the sounds of the likes of Buck Owens and the so-called C&W outlaws, Merle Haggard and Waylon Jennings (and, by extension, Dwight Yoakam). There are still plenty of pick-up trucks, dirt roads, and bars in and around Bakersfield if you want to stay in touch with your black-hat wearing outlaw side while working on your graduate degree.

University of California College of Medicine, Irvine

UCLA School of Medicine, Los Angeles

University of Southern California School of Medicine, Los Angeles

Loma Linda University School of Medicine, Loma Linda

Western University of Health Sciences, College of Osteopathic Medicine of the Pacific, Pomona

ON THE LOLLAPALOOZA TOUR

Like a modern-day medieval market updated for cyberspace, the annual Lollapalooza Tour combines the best of alternative rock and world music with an astonishing advertising festival for every New Age practice and product in America. Get your belly button pierced again, donate all your extra change to rescue some obscure environmental cause, and then go bash your brains out in the biggest mosh pit in existence. And you don't have to pack up your puppy or jump in a day-glo painted van like Phish or the Deadheads. Stand still one summer and the Lollapalooza will drop in on you. Here are the schools on the Lollapalooza Tour:

Seattle

University of Washington School of Medicine

Denver

University of Colorado School of Medicine

Kansas City

University of Missouri, Kansas City School of Medicine

University of Health Sciences College of Osteopathic Medicine, Kansas City

St. Louis

St. Louis University Health Sciences Center

Washington University School of Medicine, St. Louis

Indianapolis

Indiana University School of Medicine

Columbus

Ohio State University College of Medicine

Chicago

University of Chicago, Pritzker School of Medicine

Finch University of Health Sciences, Chicago Medical School

University of Illinois College of Medicine

Loyola University, Chicago Stritch School of Medicine

Northwestern University Medical School

Rush Medical College of Rush University

Detroit

Wayne State University School of Medicine

Boston

Harvard Medical School, Cambridge

Boston University School of Medicine

Tufts University School of Medicine

Philadelphia

Thomas Jefferson University, Jefferson Medical College, Philadelphia

Medical College of Pennsylvania and Hahnemann University School of Medicine, Philadelphia

University of Pennsylvania School of Medicine, Philadelphia

Temple University School of Medicine, Philadelphia

Philadelphia College of Osteopathic Medicine, Philadelphia

Pittsburgh

Pennsylvania State University College of Medicine, Hershey

University of Pittsburgh School of Medicine

Lake Erie College of Osteopathic Medicine, Erie

New York City

Yeshiva University, Albert Einstein College of Medicine, Bronx

Columbia University College of Physicians and Surgeons

Cornell University Medical College

Mount Sinai School of Medicine of the City University of New York

New York University School of Medicine

New York Medical College, Valhalla

SUNY Health Science Center at Brooklyn College of Medicine

SUNY Stony Brook School of Medicine Health Sciences Center

New York Institute of Technology College of Osteopathic Medicine, Old Westbury

Atlanta

Emory University School of Medicine, Atlanta

Morehouse School of Medicine, Atlanta

Medical College of Georgia School of Medicine, Augusta

Mercer University School of Medicine, Macon

Raleigh

Bowman Gray School of Medicine of Wake Forest University, Winston-Salem

Duke University School of Medicine, Durham

University of North Carolina at Chapel Hill School of Medicine

East Carolina University School of Medicine, Greenville

Austin

Baylor College of Medicine, Houston

University of Texas Houston Medical School

University of Texas Medical School at Galveston

Texas A&M University Health Science Center, College Station

University of Texas Medical School at San Antonio

Dallas

Texas Tech University Health Science Center School of Medicine, Lubbock

University of Texas Southwestern Medical Center at Dallas

University of North Texas Health Science Center College of
Osteopathic Medicine, Fort Worth

Phoenix

Midwest University Arizona College of Osteopathic Medicine, Glendale

University of Arizona College of Medicine, Tucson

Los Angeles

University of California College of Medicine, Irvine

UCLA School of Medicine, Los Angeles

University of Southern California School of Medicine, Los Angeles

Loma Linda University School of Medicine, Loma Linda

Western University of Health Sciences College of Osteopathic
Medicine of the Pacific, Pomona

Sacramento

University of California School of Medicine, Davis

San Francisco

University of California School of Medicine, San Francisco

MUST-SEE CLASSIC
FILMS FOR FUTURE DOCTORS

Here's an international selection of classic movies about the practice of medicine—well, at least a lot of them have the word *doctor* in the title. Just remember that if you want to see good doctors performing public service, medical miracles, and acts of mercy, you'll generally have to stick to TV. But if you can take the celluloid elbow poking you in the ribs, these films can be lots of fun. Want to have a great all-night party for your fellow resident students in the basement of the hospital? Get your hands on as many of the Dr. Jekyll and Mr. Hyde films as you can and stage a minimarathon.

The Cabinet of Dr. Caligari (1919). You might as well get used to it right up front: Like many cinematic doctors, Caligari is portrayed as a maniac. Or is he? This film is the prototype for droves of flicks in both the film noir and horror genres. It may be almost 100 years old, but it will still give you the willies.

Dr. Jekyll and Mr. Hyde (1931). This was the first and the best adaptation of the Robert Louis Stevenson novel about the good doctor with an assertive evil half. It stars Fredrick March and Miriam Hopkins.

Dr. Erlich's Magic Bullet (1940). Edward G. Robinson portrays the German doctor, Paul Erlich, who discovered Serum 606, the first cure for syphilis. Robinson might seem out of character, since his usual role was venting guys with a Tommy gun, but he gives a marvelously humane performance. The movie also stars a very young Ruth Gordon.

Dr. Jekyll and Mr. Hyde (1941). This is the second version and it can generally be rated number two in every category but casting. The film stars Spencer Tracy and a very fetching Ingrid Bergman.

Doctor in the House (1954). This was the first movie in a long series of British doctor movies starring the distinguished Dirk Bogard. Other titles included *Doctor at Sea, Doctor at Large,* and *Doctor in Distress.* The first is considered the best of them all, and the story follows the lives of four medical students working their way through years of study.

Dr. No (1962). Okay, so it's a spy film, not a doctor film. But it's the first James Bond movie, and it's great. The sinister and quite scrutable Dr. No—played by Bernard Lee—is strictly into bad medicine for the entire Western World. His vicious inventions—including those super-powerful but weird rubber-gloved hands—and his flirtation with radiation make him the archetypal bad guy of the Techno Age. Add to these the bonuses that you get the one-and-only "real" Bond in the young Sean Connery, and that the film features Ursula Andress.

Dr. Strangelove, or How I Learned to Stop Worrying and Love the Bomb (1963). This film has absolutely nothing to do with medicine, but it is the best black comedy you'll ever see. Director Stanley Kubrick's masterpiece is about an incipient nuclear holocaust urged into existence by the mysterious doctor. It features the inimitable comic talent of Peter Sellars in a dual role (one of which is the demented Strangelove), as well as hilarious performances by George C. Scott, Sterling Hayden, Slim Pickens, and Keenan Wynn as Col. Batguano. This is the anti–*Dr. No*, and they make a great double feature for the right crowd of sleep-deprived medical students.

Dr. Doolittle (1967). English country doctor Rex Harrison discovers that with a little tutoring from his pet Macaw, he can talk to the animals. This leads to a flirtation with a seal, vegetarianism, and a flight to the moon on the back of a giant moth. The cast is studded with human stars—including Samantha Eggar, Richard Attenborough, and Anthony Newley—all upstaged by a "Pushmi-Pullyu," a two-headed, dancing llama.

M*A*S*H* (1970). Donald Sutherland, Elliot Gould, Robert Duvall, and Sally Kellerman star in this excellent triage-as-laugh-riot film about medics working near the front during the Korean War. The Robert Altman movie is scalpel-sharp and lent some of this edge to the forever-running TV series with Alan Alda and company.

The Hospital (1971). George C. Scott stars as a doc caught in a terminally mismanaged hospital—you may have come across some of the macabre jokes in your own experience. The screenplay by Paddy

Chayefsky is very funny in a dark, dark way. Diana Rigg is lovely, and Frances Sternhagen does a virtuoso turn as the nurse from hell.

Dr. Butcher, M.D. (1979). "Dr. Butcher loves New York. There are so many victims!" This film proves that the Italians can make a horror film just as bad as anything produced in Hollywood and for half the price. It's all downhill after the title, but the campy acting and dizzy story can be very entertaining. Best viewed with the sound turned off and you and your friends inventing impromptu dialogue.

Dr. Heckyl and Mr. Hype (1980). Here's a horror film spoof that's actually funny. A hideously deformed podiatrist quaffs down a snake oil elixir and is transformed into Oliver Reed. Upon seeing his new self in the mirror, the doctor proclaims, "Good God! I'm beautiful!" Jackie Coogan plays Sergeant Fleacollar, the desk clerk at the neighborhood nick.

Flatliners (1987). Keifer Sutherland, Julia Roberts, and Kevin Bacon star in this cult classic about medical students who play games with the doctor's ultimate enemy—death. They should know better.

Dead Ringers (1988). Horror master David Cronenberg's tale of twin brother doctors from Toronto locked inside a drug nightmare features Jeremy Irons in a brilliant dual performance. It's one thing to make a really creepy movie, but to make a horror film that includes great acting is special. Don't miss this one.

Article 99 (1991). Keifer Sutherland is back in the hospital again, this time with Ken Allotta. There is terrible corruption and neglect at a veteran's hospital. Some fine performances highlight this gritty look inside a crumbling public institution.

Awakenings (1991). Robert DeNiro looks remarkably fit for a guy who wakes up from a coma he's been in for decades. Based on a true story, the film depicts the temporary cure for a rare disease that allows this rebirth. Then as the young doctor, played by Robin Williams, looks on, his friend and patient returns to his deep sleep as the effects of the wonder drug wear off. A bittersweet movie and a bit of a tearjerker, but well worth watching.

YOUR FUTURE

"Health is wholeness and balance, an inner resilience that allows you to meet the demands of living without being overwhelmed . . . .Whenever the equilibrium of the body breaks down, your healing system attempts to reestablish it. When you cut your finger, for example, you do not have to pray for the cut to heal or seek out a finger healer. As long as the wound is clean, and no underlying chronic illness is present, the cut heals by itself. That is an example of spontaneous healing, mediated by the healing system . . .

"Human beings are bodies, minds, and spirits. Health necessarily involves all those components, and any program intended to improve health must address all of them. Conventional medicine pays almost exclusive attention to our physical bodies, giving lip service to our minds, but not really taking them seriously, and totally ignoring our spirits. In spite of a great deal of research demonstrating the causative role of stress in illness and the interplay of emotions and immunity, most medical researchers and practitioners assume that physical causes can explain all diseases and that physical treatments—drugs usually—are the only ones that count."

Andrew Weil, M.D.
8 Weeks to Optimum Health
Knopf, 1997

Face it. Going to medical school isn't about "now," it's all about "later." At this point, you are the "before" picture, with oily skin, hair that wilts, a cheap suit, warts, and bitten fingernails. You jump into the M.D. machine and disappear for a bunch of years. Once you graduate, you'll expect to be the "after" picture—tall, tailored, pimple free, respected, and rich. You hope to be a beacon of comfort to the sick, a staunch pillar of the community, the owner of a five-bedroom, red-brick, Georgian mansion in a security-controlled, country-club setting. Despite what you've been led to believe by the institutionalized, overworked American Dream, education can take you only so far, and then you better have some talent or one heck of an inheritance coming. The medical profession has changed radically in recent years, and your sheepskin is no longer a free ticket to paradise. However, the final outcome of your dream is less likely to take on nightmarish proportions if you pick the right school in the right place. Remember that there are no guarantees. Malpractice insurance is insanely expensive, whether you graduate from Harvard or Rah!-Rah! State Kindergarten of Medicine. Don't go out and buy that new set of Ping golf clubs until you've checked out the lists in this chapter.

HIGHEST AVERAGE STUDENT LOAN DEBT

"I owe, I owe, so off to work I go!" There you'll be back in the cold, cruel world, with your stethoscope, a pre-owned EKG monitor, a shiny, new medical license, high hopes . . . and a student loan bill of $70,000 or more—much more—to pay off. These guys don't want to wait for their money, either. Maybe you'd better take that offer as junior slave in a partnership, or the administrative grind back at the hospital where you served your residency. You'll need the steady income. Here are the medical schools whose students incur the highest debt for their education.

Kirksville College of Osteopathic Medicine, Kirksville, MO	$124,999
Lake Erie College of Osteopathic Medicine, Erie, PA	$120,000

Philadelphia College of Osteopathic Medicine, Philadelphia, PA	$119,000
Nova Southeastern University College of Medicine, Miami, FL	$118,498
University of Osteopathic Medicine and Health Sciences, Des Moines, IA	$112,000
University of Health Sciences College of Osteopathic Medicine, Kansas City, MO	$109,000
Temple University School of Medicine, Philadelphia, PA	$105,000
Georgetown University School of Medicine, Washington, DC	$99,000
Rush Medical College at Rush University, Chicago, IL	$98,000
University of Vermont School of Medicine, Burlington, VT	$95,000
Jefferson Medical College Thomas Jefferson University, Philadelphia, PA	$94,207
UCLA School of Medicine, Los Angeles, CA	$93,000
Morehouse College School of Medicine, Atlanta, GA	$91,146
Midwestern University Chicago College of Osteopathic Medicine, Chicago, IL	$90,221
University of Miami School of Medicine, Miami, FL	$87,525
Mt. Sinai School of Medicine, New York, NY	$87,000
Northwestern University Medical School, Chicago, IL	$86,050
Virginia Commonwealth University Medical College, Richmond, VA	$84,000
Tulane University School of Medicine, New Orleans, LA	$83,581
Pennsylvania State University College of Medicine, Hershey, PA	$83,023
Eastern Virginia Medical College of the Medical School of Hampton Roads, Norfolk, VA	$83,000
University of Pittsburgh School of Medicine, Pittsburgh, PA	$80,000
Case Western Reserve University School of Medicine, Cleveland, OH	$79,000
University of Colorado School of Medicine, Denver, CO	$75,195

SCHOOLS WITH
NOBEL PRIZE WINNERS AS ALUMNI

The Nobel Memorial Prize in Physiology and Medicine has been award-ed annually since 1901, but there were very few Americans who won in the early years. However, in the last 50 years, doctors and scientists in the United States have dominated the in this category. Not every winner is a medical doctor, but all the winners have been thrown onto the list anyway to give you an idea of how your school stacks up. Columbia and Johns Hopkins are tied for second place with six winners each, and Harvard wins hands-down with 11 graduates on this Nobel Prize win-ners list, the vast majority of them medical doctors. So if you want to win a free trip to Sweden to pick up your award, you'll probably have to live in Boston.

1933   T. H. Morgan. State College of Kentucky, B.S.; Johns Hopkins University, M.D., Ph.D.

1934   George R. Minot. Harvard University, M.D., Ph.D.

William P. Murphy. Harvard University, M.A., M.D.

G. H. Whipple. Johns Hopkins University, M.D.

1943   Edward A. Doisy. University of Illinois, A. B.; Harvard University, M.A., Ph.D.

1944   Joseph Erlanger. University of California, B.S.; Johns Hopkins University, M.D.

Herbert S. Gasse. University of Wisconsin, M.A.; Johns Hopkins University, M.D.

1946   Herman J. Muller. Columbia University, B.A., M.A., M.D.

1950   Philip S. Hench. University of Pittsburgh, M.A., M.D.

Edward C. Kendall. Columbia University, M.S., Ph.D.

1952   Selman A. Waksman. Rutgers University B.Sc., M.Sc.;
       University of California, Ph.D.

1954   J. F. Enders. Yale University, A.B.; Harvard University,
       M.A., Ph.D.

       Frederick C. Robbins. Harvard University, M.A., M.D.

       Thomas H. Weller. University of Michigan, M.S.; Harvard
       University, M.D.

1956   Dickinson W. Richards, Jr. Columbia University, M.A., M.D.

1958   George W. Beadle. University of Nebraska, B.S.; Cornell
       University, M.D.

       Joshua Lederberg. Columbia University, Ph.D.

       Edward L. Tatum. University of Wisconsin, A.B., M.A., M.D.

1959   Arthur Kornberg. University of Rochester, M.D.

1962   James D. Watson. Indiana University, Ph.D.

1966   Charles B. Huggins. Harvard University, M.A., M.D.

       Peyton F. Rous. Johns Hopkins University, M.D.

1967   Halden Keffer Hartline. Lafayette College B.S.; Johns Hopkins
       University, M.D.

       George Wald. New York University, B.S.; Columbia University,
       M.A., M.D.

1968   Robert W. Holley. University of Illinois, A.B.; Cornell
       University, Ph.D.

1969   Alfred D. Hershey. Michigan State University, B.S., Ph.D.

1970   Julius Axelrod. City College of New York, B.S.; New York
        University, M.A.; George Washington University, Ph.D.

1971   Earl W. Sutherland Jr. Washington University, Ph.D.

1972   George M. Edelman. University of Pennsylvania, Ph.D.

1975   David Baltimore. Rockefeller University Ph.D.

        Howard Temin. Swarthmore College, B.A., California Institute
        of Technology, Ph.D.

1976   Baruch S. Blumberg. Columbia University, M.D.

        Daniel Carlton Gajdusek. University of Rochester, B.S.;
        Harvard University, M.A., M.D.

1977   Rosalyn S. Yalow. University of Illinois, M.S., Ph.D.

1978   Daniel Nathans. University of Missouri, M.D.

        Hamilton O. Smith. Johns Hopkins University, M.D.

1980   Baruj Benacerraf. Columbia University, B.S.; Medical College
        of Virginia, M.D.

        George Snell. Harvard University, M.A., Ph.D.

1981   Roger W. Sperry. Oberlin College, M.A.; University of
        Chicago Ph.D.

1983   Barbara McClintock. Cornell University, B.S., M.A., Ph.D.

1985   Michael S. Brown. University of Pennsylvania, B.A., M.D.

1989   J. Michael Bishop. Harvard University, M.A., M.D.

Harold Eliot Varmus. Amherst College, M.A.; Harvard University, M.A., Columbia University M.D.

1990   Joseph E. Murray. Harvard University, M.A., M.D.

Edward Donnall Thomas. University of Texas, M.A.; Harvard University, M.A., M.D.

1992   Edwin G. Krebs. Washington University, M.D.

1993   Phillip Allen Sharp. University of Illinois, Ph.D.

1994   Alfred G. Gilman. Case Western Reserve University, M.D., Ph.D.

Martin Rodbell. Johns Hopkins University, M.D.; University of Washington, Ph.D.

1995   Edwin B. Lewis. California Institute of Technology, Ph.D.

Eric F. Weischaus. University of Notre Dame B.S.; Yale University, Ph.D.

SCHOOLS WITH NATIONAL
MEDAL OF SCIENCE WINNERS

Established in 1962, the National Medal of Science is bestowed on winners by the president of the United States for outstanding achievement in physical, biological, mathematical, engineering, behavioral, or social sciences. It is not handed out annually; you've got to really do something special and get the attention of the people in the White House to get this one. This award makes an excellent warm-up for—or consolation for not receiving—the un-American Nobel Prize. The medal itself shows a human figure surrounded by earth, sea, and sky, seeking to comprehend nature (made in America). Here are the winners in disciplines related to medicine who graduated from institutions with medical school affiliations—some of them are even doctors.

1994   Elizabeth Neufeld. Biochemistry. University of California, Los Angeles

1993   Daniel Nathans. Biology. Johns Hopkins University

Salome G. Waelsch. Biology. Yeshiva University, Albert Einstein School of Medicine

1992   Eleanor J. Gibson. Psychology. Cornell University

Howard M. Temin. Biology. University of Wisconsin (McArdle Laboratory for Cancer Research)

1991   Mary Ellen Avery. Medicine. Harvard Medical School

1990   Elkan R. Blount. Medicine. Harvard School of Public Health

Kay Folkers. Biochemistry. University of Texas (Institute for Biomedical Research)

1989   Viktor Hamburger. Biology. Washington University

Philip Leder. Biochemistry. Harvard Medical School

Harden M. McConnell. Biochemistry. Stanford University

1988   Konrad E. Bloch. Medicine. Harvard Medical School

Micheal S. Brown. Medicine. University of Texas Medical School

Joseph L. Goldstein. Medicine University of Texas Medical School

1987   Harry Eagle. Biology. Yeshiva University Albert Einstein College of Medicine

William S. Johnson. Biochemistry. Stanford University

Paul C. Lauterbur. Medical University of Illinois

1986   Stanley Cohen. Biochemistry. Vanderbilt University

Donald A. Henderson. Medicine. Johns Hopkins University School of Medicine

George A. Palade. Biology. Yale University

1985   Paul Berg. Biology. Stanford University

Wendell L. Roelofs. Biology. Cornell University

1979   Arthur Kornberg. Biochemistry. Stanford University

Ledyard Stebbins. Genetics. University of California, Davis

1976   Keith R. Porter. Biology. University of Colorado

Efrain Racker. Biochemistry. Cornell University

1975   Hallowell Davis. Medicine. Washington University

Paul Gyorgy. Pediatrics. University of Pennsylvania

1974   James V. Neel. Genetics. University of Michigan

1973   Earl W. Sutherland. Biochemistry. University of Miami

Erwin Chargaff. Biochemistry. Columbia University

1968   B. F. Skinner. Psychology. Harvard University

1967   Harry F. Harlow. Psychology. University of Wisconsin

Michael Heidelberger. Immunology. New York University

1966   Sewell Wright. Genetics. University of Wisconsin

1964   Neal Elgar Miller. Psychology. Harvard University

SCHOOLS WITH GRADUATES AT THE MAYO CLINIC

The Mayo Clinic is perhaps the most esteemed medical care institution in America. As such, it attracts many of the best medical specialists in the world. If you aspire to this top rank of doctors, perhaps you should look into the schools where these men and women trained. Here are some of the most prominent among this closely knit group of talented physicians along with their alma maters.

Dr. Richard Bryan (Orthopedic surgery), Northwestern University School of Medicine

Dr Philip Bernatz (Thoracic surgery), University of Maryland School of Medicine

Dr. Thomas Bunch (Rheumatology), Northwestern University School of Medicine

Dr. Robert Frye (Cardiology), Vanderbilt University School of Medicine

Dr. William Furlow (Urology), George Washington University School of Medicine

Dr. Clark Hoagland (Hematology; head of bone marrow transplant unit), University of Virginia School of Medicine

Dr. Keith Kelly (Surgery; gastroenterologist), University of Tennessee School of Medicine

Dr. Patrick Kelly (Neurosurgery; specialist in brain tumors), SUNY Medical School

Dr. Robert Kyle (Oncology; specialist in myeloma), Northwestern University School of Medicine

Dr. Edward Laws (Neurosurgery), Johns Hopkins University School of Medicine

Dr. W. Spencer Payne (Thoracic surgery), St. Louis University School of Medicine

Dr. Harold Perry (Dermatology, specializing in skin growths for burn victims), University of Minnesota Medical School

Dr. Mark Pittelkow (Dermatology, specializing in skin growth for burn victims), Mayo Medical School

Dr. Douglas Pritchard (Orthopedic surgery), Tufts University School of Medicine

Dr. Charles Reed (Chairman of Allergic Diseases program), Columbia University School of Physicians and Surgeons

Dr. David Utz (Urologist; specialist in prostate cancer), Mayo Medical School

Dr. Jack Whisant (Neurology, particularly cerebrovascular disorders), University of Arkansas for Medical Sciences College of Medicine

Dr. John Wood (Plastic surgery), Case Western Reserve University School of Medicine

SCHOOLS WITH GRADUATES AT NATIONAL INSTITUTE OF HEALTH AGENCIES

One thing about a medical degree—it's good enough for government work. Department heads in various sectors of the national health care services come from a wide-ranging array of medical schools. The only schools with two graduates in federal health care management are the University of Mississippi Medical School, Jackson, MS, and Meharry School of Medicine in Nashville, TN.

Center For Disease Control and Prevention: David Satcher, Case Western Reserve School of Medicine

Office of Disease Prevention and Health Promotion: Claude E. Fox, University of Mississippi School of Medicine

National Center for Environmental Health: Richard J. Jackson, University of California Medical School, San Francisco

National Center for Infectious Diseases: James M. Hughes, Stanford University Medical School

Center For Drug Evaluation and Research: Janet Woodcock, Northwestern University School of Medicine

Maternal and Child Health Bureau: Audrey H. Nora, University of Mississippi School of Medicine

Bureau of Primary Health Care: Marilyn H. Gaston, University of Cincinnati College of Medicine

National Institute of Health: Harold E. Varmus, Columbia University College of Physicians and Surgeons

National Eye Institute: Carl Kupfer, Johns Hopkins University School of Medicine

National Heart, Lung and Blood Institute: Claude J. M. L'enfant; Dr. L'enfant graduated the University of Paris Medical School in 1956. He became a naturalized American citizen in 1965, and for his illustrious career work was awarded an honorary degree at the State University of New York in 1988.

National Institute of Arthritis and Skin Diseases: Stephan I. Katz, Tulane University School of Medicine (Arthritis and skin disease)

Secretary of the Department of Health and Human Services: Donna E. Shalala, Meharry Medical College. This is a big political job, and Dr. Shalala is probably back in private practice by now, for which reason we list her probable successor:

Assistant Secretary of the Department of Health and Human Services: Phillip R. Lee, Stanford University School of Medicine

DOCTORS WHO SCRIBBLE

Doctors Who Became Authors

Medical students have extensive training in writing—in English and Latin, ad nauseum. Then they get out into medical practice, and it's more writing—tons of prescriptions, research papers. Ah, sometimes saving the world gets old. You could try saving the second mortgage instead, and a popular way among physicians to do that is by writing a book. There is a long, rich tradition of doctor authors. Here are a few.

Anton Chekhov. Chekhov began his short life (he died at age 44) as a medical doctor, but soon segued into a second career as one of the masters of the short story, as well as a world-class playwright. His plays like *The Cherry Orchard, The Seagull,* and *Uncle Vanya* are still in production, from high school gymnasiums to Broadway. Chekhov's short stories, for example "Lady With Lapdog," "Ward Six," and "The Darling," demonstrate his amazing ability to compress an entire lifetime into a few crystal-clear pages.

Louis-Ferdinand Celine. Born Louis-Ferdinand Destouches, he wrote masterpieces of black humour—*Journey to the End of the Night* and *Death on the Installment Plan,* under the adopted name of Celine. Celine began his career as a physician treating the Parisian poor, a clientele he wrote about as "a bunch of crumbs." However, he treated them for free. "They didn't have any money anyway," he explained. Celine died in 1961. Today he is widely admired for his unique style, combining elegant prose with street slang to hilarious effect. He is also despised for being a Nazi collaborator and anti-Semitic pamphleteer, unrepentant in old age. Celine kept this dark side out of his novels, which have inspired many modern American writers. Before he died, the poet Allen Ginsberg and author William Burroughs visited Celine in France. They found a garrulous old man, still railing against Jewish plots. Ginsberg rose and shrugged: "Nevertheless, sir, we salute you as the greatest French prose writer of the 20th century." Unfortunately, that was not all he was.

Michael Crichton. Scientists laughed when they read *Jurassic Park,* the tale of the mighty *Tyrannosaurus rex* resurrected from tiny strands of DNA. Of course, by then, Crichton, Steven Spielberg, and company were laughing all the way to the bank. But as it turns out, scientists have recently found a few bugs preserved in amber for a few million years, and are making noises about extracting their DNA, and . . . The point is, Doc Mike might be right about raising the dead with DNA, but instead of publishing a research paper and having jealous scientists tear it apart for free, he wrote a book and let jealous editors tear it apart for big bucks. Now instead of having to worry about a thieving colleague's claim that he made the discovery first, all Crichton has to deal with is whether a thieving publisher is cheating him on the royalties. What makes more sense to you? We thought so.

Dr. Benjamin Spock. We're not talking about the emotionless but like-able, pointy-eared extraterrestrial from *Star Trek,* but the likeable, kind-ly looking old pediatrician told our parents how to raise us through his multimillion selling books. Don't blame your parents if you feel you turned out bad—they were only following orders from that tall drink of water, Spock. Thanks a lot, Doc.

Dr. Pritikin, Dr. Susan Love, Dr. Andrew Weil, Dr. Robert Atkins, and company. As the fattening of the nation continues, one thing remains constant: Americans will do anything to lose weight except eat less. Ergo, the sure way to get a book on the bestseller list is to slap a "Doctor" in front of your name and dream up a diet. Doesn't much matter what the diet is—The Miracle-Beer-and-Potato-Chips Diet, The All-Kidney-Bean-High-Fiber Diet. Count on it, people will buy the book.

Dr. Joyce Brothers. Doctor Brothers may be sanest person in America, but good God almighty, the woman is dull. Five minutes of her advice could put a manic speed freak in a torpor. Let's say you get through medical school and residency as sane as Doctor Brothers appears to be. It's nearly impossible, but let's say it happened. One thing for sure: You will have already seen enough affliction to last six lifetimes. Why not apply your terminal sanity towards lulling the savage beasts you know are lurking out there via books, talk shows, and commercials? They'll show you the money, don't worry about that! After all, Doctor B's getting on in years now, and soon she's sure to stop making sense. *Someone* has got to jump into the breach. Why couldn't it be you?

WHERE THE LIVING IS EASY

Schools in Areas with the Lowest Cost of Living

Let's say you don't manage to win the Nobel Prize or the National Medal of Science. Maybe you don't get a job at the Mayo Clinic or even with the feds in your first year out of school. Let's say you don't get invited to join a great partnership of established doctors, and you owe so much money in student loans that you don't have the cash to rent an office to start your own practice. Maybe you'd like to own a car, live in a reasonably nice environment, and eat three meals a day most days of the year. You're going to want to be able to stretch those dollars, so it would be a good idea to live where the cost of living is low. If you graduate from a school in this area, the cost of maintaining life during school will be much lower, perhaps lowering your indebtedness upon graduating. You might also have a better chance of getting and keeping a job, since the local employers will see you as a hometown boy or girl. The government factors in the costs of food, beverage, housing, apparel, transportation, medical care, fuel, utilities, and entertainment in a certain geographic area to come up with the Consumer Price Index. The average for American cities is 148.2. Here are the areas in the United States with the lowest cost of living, as measured by the Consumer Price Index, and the schools nearby.

1. Tampa–St. Petersburg-Clearwater, FL   126.5
   This is the cheapest place to live in America today, and the sunshine is free. Contrary to popular belief, there are people under
   the age of 65 living in this area—maybe not in St. Petersburg, but
   certainly in Tampa.

   University of South Florida College of Medicine, Tampa, FL

2. New Orleans, LA   129
   The fish are jumping and the cotton is high in the Big Easy. You
   have to use a machete to cut your way through the summer
   humidity, and life expectancy is marred somewhat by Louisiana's
   murder rate—the highest per capita rate in the nation—but survival is cheap if you don't weaken. However, fun is readily available, and can cost you plenty in large quantities.

   Louisiana State University School of Medicine in New Orleans

   Tulane University School of Medicine, New Orleans

   Louisiana State University School of Medicine in Shreveport

3. Houston-Galveston-Brazoria, TX   137.9
   So, it's flat, it's humid, it's industrial. But the Tex-Mex food is
   great, you can get Lone Star and Tecate, the Gulf shore beaches of
   Padre Island are reasonably close by, the rush hour traffic is truly
   exciting (the highways are bumper to bumper, but everybody is
   still going 100 m.p.h.), and the price index is right.

   Baylor College of Medicine, Houston

   University of Texas Houston Medical School

   University of Texas Medical School at Galveston

5. Dallas–Fort Worth, TX   141.2
   This is the Cowboy and Cowgirl Heaven of Texas. If you don't
   believe it, ask any Dallasite, who will be happy to confirm this
   information. They have been a little lax with their zoning laws
   though. It's not unusual to find 35-story, high-rise office buildings
   sprouting up in the middle of suburban tract housing. But this

same loose attitude can be a boon if you want to keep your favorite quarter horse in the backyard. There are plenty of neighborhoods in which horses are second only to dogs as pets.

University of Texas Southwestern Medical Center at Dallas

University of North Texas Health Science Center College of Osteopathic Medicine, Fort Worth

6. Kansas City–St. Louis, MO   141.3
Kansas City has been the central marketplace between the Midwest and the Southwest for hundreds of years. The city rises in steps built on bluffs along the banks of the Kansas and Missouri Rivers. St. Louis is a hub of America's inland waterways with its command of the Mississippi River. The 630-foot high Gateway Arch towers over one of the most successful urban renewal projects in the nation. These are cities of industry, agriculture, and transportation. Think of them this way: Missouri is just California without an ocean.

St. Louis University Health Sciences Center

Washington University School of Medicine, St. Louis

University of Missouri, Columbia School of Medicine

University of Missouri, Kansas City School of Medicine

University of Health Sciences College of Osteopathic Medicine, Kansas City

7. Cincinnati-Hamilton, OH   142.4
This is a conservative city. They closed down the Robert Mapplethorpe photography exhibition in a heartbeat, and it's almost impossible to find *Playboy* magazine on the newsstands here. Maybe you think that's all good. Draped over rolling hills on the banks of the Ohio River, Cincinnati is one of the most scenic towns in the Midwest, plus it's just across the river from Covington and Newport, KY, the wild and woolly towns that play Mr. Hyde to Cincinnati's Dr. Jekyll.

University of Cincinnati College of Medicine

8. Miami–Fort Lauderdale, FL   143.6
    Come so deep South it doesn't even seem southern anymore.
    What you save on clothes you'll invest in sunscreen to keep those
    parts of your body that have never seen the sun from getting
    burned. There are low prices and low wages here, but the Gulf
    Stream and café Cubano make it all worthwhile. You could starve
    to death in much worse places.

    University of Miami School of Medicine, Miami

    Nova Southeastern University College of Osteopathic Medicine,
    Fort Lauderdale

9. Minneapolis–St. Paul, MN   143.6
    Although these cities and the Miami region have the same
    Consumer Price Index, Minneapolis–St. Paul has snow instead of
    sunshine and no mountain nearby to offset this disadvantage with
    skiing, so they drop to Number 9. But Minnesota is the Land of
    Sky Blue Waters, and the population has set aside more millions of
    acres for game refuges than any other state. It's also the home of
    Control Data, 3M, Honeywell, General Mills, Pillsbury, and Land
    O' Lakes. Don't knock it until you've tried it.

    University of Minnesota Medical School, Minneapolis

10. Detroit, MI   144
    There are still blocks in downtown Detroit where you can buy a
    sagging wreck of an inner city house for less than a used car, but
    the Motor City is coming back to life after more than ten years of
    blight and destruction. Backed by a federally financed "empower-
    ment zone" on the site of an abandoned 55-acre Cadillac plant,
    minority-owned auto part suppliers are providing jobs for a
    neighborhood that has seen 50 percent unemployment statistics
    for many years. Perhaps you can help put the heart back into one
    of the greatest industrial cities in the world.

    Wayne State University School of Medicine

NEAR THE JOBS

If you want your career to take off like you were shot out of a cannon, then go to school where the economy is predicted to be booming by the time you graduate. This is a list of the metropolitan areas with the highest projected growth in jobs by the year 2015. Get to where the action is going to be, and stick in there. It's not a bad idea to pair up the cities that appear both here and on the lowest cost of living list. Here's a hint: Dallas, Houston, Minneapolis, Tampa.

	New Jobs Expected
Atlanta, GA	1.4 million

    Emory University School of Medicine, Atlanta

    Morehouse School of Medicine, Atlanta

Washington, DC and vicinity	1.3 million

    George Washington University School of Medicine and Health Sciences

    Georgetown University School of Medicine

    Howard University College of Medicine

    Uniformed Services University of the Health Sciences, Bethesda

Los Angeles–Long Beach, CA	1.2 million

    UCLA School of Medicine, Los Angeles

    University of Southern California School of Medicine, Los Angeles

Houston, TX	1.2 Million

    Baylor College of Medicine, Houston

    University of Texas Houston Medical School

    University of Texas Medical School at Galveston

Dallas, TX	1.1 million
University of Texas Southwestern Medical Center at Dallas	
University of North Texas Health Science Center College of Osteopathic Medicine, Fort Worth	
Orange County, CA	1 million
University of California College of Medicine, Irvine	
Seattle, WA	890,000
University of Washington School of Medicine	
San Diego, CA	870,000
University of California School of Medicine, San Diego	
Minneapolis–St. Paul, MN	750,000
Mayo Medical School, Rochester	
University of Minnesota, Duluth School of Medicine	
University of Minnesota Medical School, Minneapolis	
Tampa–St. Petersburg-Clearwater, FL	714,000
University of South Florida College of Medicine, Tampa	

JUST IN CASE

If there's one thing they teach you in medical school, it is to plan for every contingency. There you are, happily working your socks off, curing cancer and the common cold on a case-by-case basis, when suddenly the market is so glutted with doctors who had the same idea about making a lot of money as you that the HMO doesn't need you anymore, or the escalating cost of hospital care prices everybody out of being sick, so you have no patients anymore, or Hillary Clinton actually does get

Congress to pass a national health care bill that totally eliminates doctors. Okay, that *can't* happen to you—but just in case, here are the states that pay the highest average weekly unemployment benefits. For your protection, this list is followed by another one that documents the skinflint states that pay the least in unemployment benefits. Move if you have to.

Highest

1. Massachusetts: $217 per week. It's too bad Boston isn't in Florida. This is the kind of money you could live on if you had to.

2. Washington, DC: $213 per week. It's easy for them to pay so much, since everybody works for the government and never loses his job. Unemployment in DC just means they have to hire more people to administer the benefits, and they cancel each other out.

3. New Jersey: $207 per week. It doesn't look like much, but as long as you can get your hands on over $200, you might just make it.

4. Michigan: $204 per week. Hope for an Indian summer and a mild winter.

5. Connecticut: $201 per week. Maybe it won't pay off your student loan from Yale, but it'll keep you in Ring-Dings until you figure out a new plan.

6. Hawaii: $196 per week. Now we're talking. Assuming you sleep on the beach, you might be able to live on the weekly dole in the islands.

7. Rhode Island: $194 per week. Small state, big stipend, one school.

8. Minnesota: $190 per week. Of course, it all goes to your heating bill.

9. Pennsylvania: $189 per week. They don't pay much for liberty. You'd be better off working.

10. New York: $181 per week. Not bad for a state with more people unemployed than some states employ. New York pays out close to $2 billion in annual unemployment benefits, trailing only California, which pays an average of $50 less per week.

Lowest

1. Louisiana: $102 per week. Not a good place to get fired unless you like crayfish and know how to catch them.

2. Indiana: $107 per week. Hoosiers evidently do not believe in the free lunch.

3. Mississippi: $111 per week. You'll be living on Mississippi Mud pies.

4. Tennessee: $113 per week. Put your Ford up on blocks and move in.

5. Alabama: $116 per week. Sweat soup isn't too bad.

6. Nebraska: $120 per week. Hope you like corn on the cob. Hope you like cob, for that matter.

7. South Dakota: $120 per week. There's not much unemployment here, but then there's not all that much employment either.

8. California: $131 per week. When the promise leaves the Promised Land, you're on your own.

9. Arkansas: $133 per week. No wonder the Clintons left.

10. Arizona: $135 per week. Take your first check, buy a lizard cookbook, move out into the desert.

PHYSICIANS BY SPECIALTY AND SEX

Once you start attending medical school, you will be faced with a big decision—and we're not talking about your fall wardrobe. We're talking about your niche, the branch of medicine in which you'll specialize. As of 1996, there were over 720,000 physicians in the United States specializing in over 35 separate disciplines, ranging from aerospace medicine to urology. They are listed here with the number of men and of women who are practicing in each specialty. Pin it to the wall and throw darts at it.

	Men	Women
Aerospace Medicine	543	32
Allergy and Immunology	3,039	736

Anesthesiology	26,431	6,422
Cardiovascular Disease	17,705	1,293
Child Psychiatry	3,396	2,148
Colon/Rectal Surgery	938	52
Dermatology	6,110	2,453
Diagnostic Radiology	16,051	3,757
Emergency Medicine	15,815	3,297
Family Practice	45,176	13,934
Forensic Pathology	366	130
Gastroenterology	8,822	729
General Practice	14,507	2,362
General Preventive Medicine	870	399
General Surgery	34,268	3,302
Internal Medicine	66,432	21,810
Neurological Surgery	4,675	213
Neurology	9,230	12,165
Nuclear Medicine	1,181	254
Obstetrics–Gynecology	23,099	10,420
Occupational Medicine	2,549	482
Ophthalmology	15,237	2,227
Orthopedic Surgery	21,360	677
Otolaryngology	8,393	693
Pathology-Anatomy/Clinical	12,993	4,891
Pediatrics	23,575	20,034
Pediatric Cardiology	1,012	324
Physical Medicine/Rehabilitation	3,798	1,767
Plastic Surgery	5,015	478
Psychiatry	27,706	10,392

Public Health	1,302	458
Pulmonary Diseases	6,627	826
Radiation Oncology	2,844	786
Radiology	7,086	953
Thoracic Surgery	2,260	50
Urological Surgery	9,642	244
Other (Can you make a living as an other?)	6,196	1,111
Unspecified	5,902	2,571

WHAT IT'S GOING TO COST YOUR PATIENTS

Hospital Costs by State

They may enter a hospital in their Sunday suits, but they might leave wearing a barrel. The zooming costs of hospital care not only affects your future patients, but it's an important figure for you as well. Those heavy medical school workloads and 100+ hour residency weeks could put you in the market for a hospital bed. True, they'll probably give you an employee discount, but still . . . . The following statistics are the state-by-state average daily room charge and the average overall cost of spending a day in a hospital.

	Room Charge	Cost Per Day
Alabama	$210	$775
Alaska	$407	$1,136
Arizona	$300	$1,091
Arkansas	$170	$678
Colorado	$321	$961
Connecticut	$456	$1,058
Delaware	$385	$1,028
District of Columbia	$325	$1,201

Florida	$271	$940
Georgia	$191	$775
Hawaii	$348	$823
Idaho	$259	$659
Illinois	$300	$912
Indiana	$258	$898
Iowa	$221	$612
Kansas	$256	$666
Kentucky	$242	$703
Louisiana	$203	$875
Maine	$335	$738
Maryland	$266	$889
Massachussetts	$351	$1,036
Michigan	$337	$902
Minnesota	$282	$652
Mississippi	$167	$555
Missouri	$268	$863
Montana	$318	$481
Nebraska	$209	$626
Nevada	$251	$900
New Hampshire	$304	$976
New Jersey	$273	$829
New Mexico	$254	$1,046
New York	$339	$784
North Carolina	$220	$763
North Dakota	$230	$507
Ohio	$308	$940
Oklahoma	$220	$797

Oregon	$338	$1,053
Pennsylvania	$375	$861
Rhode Island	$342	$885
South Carolina	$212	$838
South Dakota	$208	$506
Tennessee	$182	$859
Texas	$223	$1,010
Utah	$353	$1,081
Vermont	$378	$676
Virginia	$220	$830
Washington	$334	$1,143
West Virginia	$223	$701
Wisconsin	$222	$744
Wyoming	$234	$537

YOUR FUTURE IN RESIDENCY

Once you've been accepted into a hospital for your residency, what can you expect, patient-wise? You'll spend a big stretch of time in the emergency room. Besides the Saturday night crowd who come in with their heads under their arms, courtesy of Smith and Wesson, there are about 20 ailments that will form the mainstay of your clienteles' problems. Here are the top 20 reasons for emergency room visits according to the U.S. Department of Health and Human Services.

1. Stomach and abdominal pain, cramps, and spasms
2. Chest pain and related symptoms
3. Fever
4. Headache, head pain
5. Cough

6. Injury to an upper extremity

7. Back symptoms

8. Symptoms in reference to the throat

9. Vomiting

10. Earache or ear infection

11. Pain in a nonspecific site

12. Shortness of breath

13. Injury to the head, neck, and face

14. Labored or difficult breathing

15. Laceration and cuts

16. Skin rash

17. Hand and finger symptoms

18. Neck symptoms

19. Leg symptoms

20. All other symptoms, constituting 52.8% of all visits—Good luck!

WHAT TO EXPECT IN PRIVATE PRACTICE

Of course, once you get into private practice, you'll get a much more interesting group of people and problems to deal with, right? At least they'll make appointments instead of riding in on stretchers. Here are the top 20 reasons people make a visit to the doctor's office from the U.S. Department of Health and Human Services.

1. General medical examination

2. Progress visit (to see if they got well)

3. Cough

4. Routine prenatal examination

5. Postoperative visit

6. Symptoms of the throat

7. Well baby examination

8. Depression

9. Earache or ear infection

10. Stomach pain, cramps, or spasms

11. Vision dysfunction

12. Skin rash

13. Back symptoms

14. Knee symptoms

15. Fever

16. Nasal congestion

17. Headache, head pain

18. Hypertension

19. Chest pain

20. Head cold and upper respiratory infection

ABOUT THE AUTHOR

Mark Baker is the author of eight other nonfiction books published by Simon & Schuster. Two of them, *Nam: The Vietnam War in the Words of the Men and Women Who Fought There* and *Cops: Their Lives in Their Own Words*, are bestsellers. Baker lives in New York City and is currently working on a book about U.S. district attorneys, to be published by Simon & Schuster in spring 1998. His other books include:

Women: American Women in Their Own Words
What Men Really Think
Sex Lives: A Sexual Self-Portrait of America
Bad Guys: America's Most Wanted in Their Own Words
The Insider's Book of Business School Lists
The Insider's Book of Law School Lists

come to us for the best prep

about KAPLAN

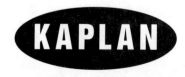

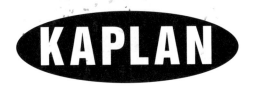

Want more information about our services, products,
or the nearest Kaplan educational center?

HERE

Call our nationwide toll-free numbers:

1-800-KAP-TEST

(for information on our live courses, private tutoring and admissions consulting)

1-800-KAP-ITEM

(for information on our products)

1-888-KAP-LOAN*

(for information on student loans)

Connect with us in cyberspace:

On **AOL**, keyword **"Kaplan"**

On the Internet's World Wide Web, open **"http://www.kaplan.com"**

Via E-mail, **"info@kaplan.com"**

Write to:

Kaplan Educational Centers
888 Seventh Avenue
New York, NY 10106

A Special Note for International Students

If you are not from the United States and need more help with the complex process of medical school admissions and information about the variety of programs available, you may be interested in Kaplan's Access America program.

Kaplan created Access America to assist students and professionals from outside the United States who want to enter the U.S. university system. Access America also has programs for obtaining professional certification in the United States. Here's a brief description of some of the help available through Access America.

The TOEFL Plus Program

At the heart of the Access America program is the intensive TOEFL Plus Academic English program. This comprehensive English course prepares students to achieve a high level of proficiency in English in order to successfully complete an academic degree. The TOEFL Plus course combines personalized instruction with guided self-study to help students gain this proficiency in a short time. Certificates of Achievement in English are awarded to certify each student's level of proficiency.

MCAT (Medical College Admissions Test) Preparation

If you plan to enter a medical school in the United States, Kaplan can help you prepare for the MCAT. Kaplan also offers professional counseling and advice to help you gain a greater understanding of the American educational system. We can help you with every step in the admissions process, from choosing the right medical school, to writing your application, to preparing for an interview.

USMLE (United States Medical Licensing Exam) and Other Medical Licensing

If you have graduated from a medical school outside the United States and would like to be certified by the Educational Commission for Foreign Medical Graduates (ECFMG) and obtain a residency in a United States Hospital, Kaplan can help you prepare for all three steps of the USMLE.

NCLEX (National Council Licensure Examination)

If you are a nurse who wishes to practice in the United States, Kaplan can help you prepare for the NCLEX or CGFNS (Commission on Graduates of Foreign Nursing Schools) exam. Kaplan can also prepare you with the English and cross-cultural knowledge that will help you become an effective nurse.

Applying to Access America

To get more information, or to apply for admission to any of Kaplan's programs for international students or professionals, you can write to us at:

Kaplan Educational Centers
International Admissions Department
888 Seventh Avenue, New York, NY 10106

Or call us at 1-800-522-7770 from within the United States, or 01-212-262-4980 outside the United States. Our fax number is 01-212-957-1654. Our E-mail address is world@kaplan.com. You can also get more information or even apply through the Internet at http://www.kaplan.com/intl.